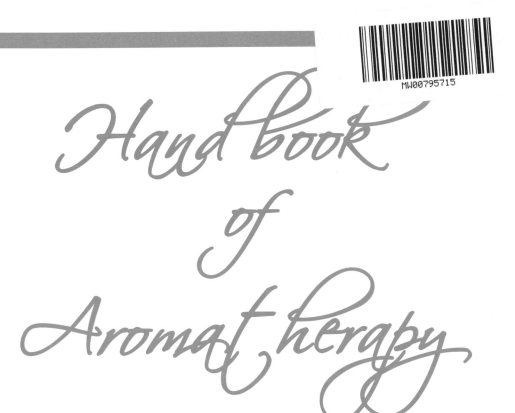

Hand book of Aromatherapy

*A complete guide to essential & carrier oils,
their application & therapeutic use for
Holistic Health & Well being*

REVISED 3RD EDITION

By
Dr. RAVI RATAN

Published by : INSTITUTE OF HOLISTIC HEALTH SCIENCES

HANDBOOK OF AROMATHERAPY

By- Dr. Ravi Ratan

First edition- 1997
Second edition- 2006
Third revised and improved edition-2009

DTP & Graphic work
Jagdeep Malhotra, Mumbai-37
jhmalhotra@yahoo.co.in

Printed by-Vishal Printers, Mumbai-37

Layout, designs and edited by-
Dr. Ravi Ratan

Published & Marketed by-
Institute of Holistic Health Sciences,
Mumbai-400037
aromatantra@yahoo.com
www.aromatantra.com

Distributed in India by-
Motilal Banarsidas Publishers Pvt. Limited,
Bunglow Road, Delhi-110007, INDIA
mlbd@vsnl.com

ISBN-978-81-208-23111-7

Price Rs. 799/-

About the author

Dr. Ratan is one of the most qualified aromatherapist in India. He achieved his Masters of Science in Zoology and later added another Masters degree in Business Administration. He belongs to a lineage of healers and teachers and thus had a great desire to be a healer. He has been in the field of manufacturing perfume and perfumery products, since more than 20 years wherein he had been dealing with the reconstituted oils, till he realized the healing potential of the natural essential oils. Aromatherapy which initially was started as a commercial venture in 1992 became his passion, wherein he worked on the healing and therapeutic 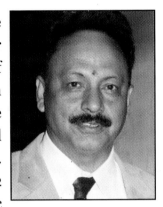 potential of various essential oils on physical as well as psychological level. Motivated by the successful results in healing and healthcare he indulged into exhaustive work on complete body therapy, which became the focal point of his thesis for D.Sc. (Medicina Alternativa), a part of this has been incorporated in this **F.M's Handbook of Aromatherapy**.

Dr. Ravi Ratan has also done extensive clinical and research work using essential oils for health and healing, specially of unhealing ulcers, wounds and sores, besides creating an aroma workout regimen for physical body, focusing on problems of each body area. Identifying causes and aromatherapy solution for the same. He has trained over a thousand beauticians, alternative therapists and health club professionals in the field of aromatherapy. In his practice of aromatherapy Dr. Ratan has combined the ancient Ayurvedic wisdom with modern aromatherapy principles- **Vedic Aromatherapy** and created various blends for health and healings. Prominent amongst these are his anointments for seven Chakras (the body's energy centers) which have been found very effective in restoring the healthy balance of mind, body, spirit. They have been used effectively by Dr. Minoo Ratan, a practicing psyco-aromatherapist and healer, for treatment of various psychosomatic disorders and other chronic conditions, her feedback on the effect had been very helpful for the efficacy of these products. Herein the fundamentals of five elements and three gunas (properties) have been used to select various essential oils for Chakra healing and balancing.

Besides providing therapies and healing including emotional release work, he has been conducting regular training programs and workshops on Aromatherapy (Basic & Advance),

Chakras & Crystals Healing and Aroma Massages with Manual Lymphatic Drainage (MLD) in India, USA, UK, Canada, Dubai & Australia. He has been approved by "National Certification Board for Therapeutic Massage & Body Work" USA to provide Continuing education hours. His training has benefitted budding aromatherapists, massage therapists, healers and other health professionals.

Dr. Ravi is well supported in his work by his wife Dr. Minoo Ratan, a Psycho aromatherapist and counselor. Both Dr. Ravi & Minoo Ratan have done extensive healing work in Vedic aromatherapy, using essential oils for Chakras energizing and harmonizing. Together they have authored "JOURNEY THROUGH CHAKRAS" a colorful informatory book on Chakras and its associated attributed explained in detail along with process of disease and healing methods. Dr. Ravi & Minoo Ratan have presented aromatherapy in various press and TV media from time to time. Dr. Ratan also patronizes FM's Aromatherapists club, having more than 1000 members. In spite of his busy schedule Dr. Ratan also provides consultancy for set up of wellness or rejuvenation centers mainly using aromatherapy in combination of other holistic therapies like Yoga, Meditation, breathing techniques, Naturopathy as a major tool, besides providing training for massage therapists and healers.

Dr. Ratan can be contacted by email at- aromatantra@yahoo.com or fmsaroma@yahoo.co.uk. Website- www.fmaromatherapy.com / www.aromatantra.com

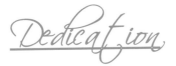

Dedication

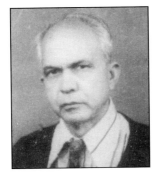

This book is dedicated to my father
Late **Dr. Sushil Kumar Sharma,**

renowned Physician and Surgeon from Muzaffarnagar, UP, India. I have always admired his healing touch and dedication to his profession, while assisting him during at his clinic during periods of extreme rush. I had seen him working on unhealing ulcers, bed sores and gangrenous wounds and wish he would have looked at the healing powers of essential oils. It is his blessing that I could use essential oils in healing all these conditions.

He had always been a source of inspiration.

Acknowledgement

I am indebted to the universal guiding principle, my Gurus (teachers) and my parents to show me the path of holistic health and healing. The knowledge of essential oils and their therapeutic effects has been revealed to me in a mysterious way. Due to early influence and upbringing in the family of medical professionals, I had always been interested in the health and health maintenance. Looking back, I feel amazed, how all the knowledge, gathered through educational ladder exposing me to Botany, Zoology and Chemistry during my graduation followed by my Masters in Zoology, and professional experience as a perfumier, got connected to the field of aromatherapy, shows the plan of the universe, to prepare me for the understanding of this subject .

The support, push and feedbacks from Minoo, my wife and a practicing psycho-armatherapist, demanding always the best possible formulations for her clients lead me to innovative combination of oils and their usage, most of it has been shared in this book. I am thankful to Minoo and my daughters Vartika and Kartikeya for their support and patience with me.

I am also thankful, to all my students and workshop participants,(most of them had been beauty or health therapists, for enriching my knowledge through various interactions. Truly, teaching is the way of learning. I also would like to offer my gratitude to all the authors, whose names are given in bibliography, as my teachers, each one has contributed to my knowledge in the field.

A book is the result of a team work, and I would like to acknowledge my co-workers, staff and graphic designers Jagdeep Malhotra and Yatin for all their time and input. I would also like to thank the distributors of this book, M/s Motilal Banarsidas Publishers Private Limited for their suggestions , feedback and support regarding the quality of the book and marketing of the same.

Table of Contents

Section-I

Section-II

Section-III

Section-IV

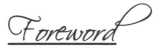

Foreword

'That which cures is medicine, That which heals is therapy'

Today the world over, alternative and complementary therapies are being re-invoked and re-established to enable mankind to regain the lost healthfulness of life. Aromatherapy is one of the most effective and safe complementary therapy, which can be used in conjunction with almost all other therapies and systems of healing. It works on us at physical, physiological and psychological levels.

Most human ailments begin in the mind. It is an established fact that psychosomatic disorders (PSD) are in fact responsible for a great share of OTC medications, mainly for stress, anxiety and depression. Psychotherapy deals in harmonizing the agonized mind while aromatherapy acts as a support system for the mind as well as the diseased physical body and physiology. Empirical studies with aromatherapy has shown, that it is most effective in increasing the body's immune level. The essential oils, used in aromatherapy are providing the necessary support to immune system and help the body to fight back. Most of the essential oils are antiseptic, antibacterial, antiviral, while some are anti-fungal, rejuvenators, hormone balancing, diuretic or with other specialized properties.

Coming from a family of medical practitioners, I had always been interested in healing aspect of the essential oils. The interest in mystical world of essential oils has grown each time they have given a result better than expected, some of my clients called miraculous results, especially for the treatment of chronic conditions like bed sores, un-healing ulcers, post operative recovery etc. Meanwhile my wife Dr. Minoo, a practicing psycho-aromatherapist, had been giving me feedbacks on various combinations / formulations done by me for her patients, mainly for the treatment of psychosomatic disorders. This third edition of the "Handbook of Aromatherapy" has got the sprinkle of not only our experience in treatment of various disorders, also from various students in the field of health and healing.

Another dimension of essential oils, I explored, had been in their use with Ayurvedic principles for healing and balancing the CHAKRAS. The Chakra anointments are created using the elements and gunas (properties) of the plants can also be used for treating physical, physiological and psychosomatic disorders. Minoo & I had been using them effectively for treating various psychosomatic as well as physiological conditions.

This book has been designed to give comprehensive knowledge and understanding of aromatherapy to the beginners as well as professionals. It has been divided into four sections; the first section covers the Materia Medica i.e. essential and carrier oils in detail, followed by a section on aromatherapy applications and methods of use. The third section is devoted to aromatic body and beauty therapy including case history taking and analyzing the conditions to be focused. For the convenience and understanding, this section covers each part of the body (head to toe) separately, to analyze the problems, causes and aromatherapy solutions for the same. Last section covers treatment of common ailments, detailed information on Evening Primrose oil (one of my favourite oils for well-being) and a ready reference guide of therapeutic uses of essential oils. Hope the readers will be able to make use of the knowledge I have tried to impart through this book.

Section-I

Understanding Aromatherapy

History of Aromatherapy

Nature of Essential Oils

How Essential Oils Works

Effect of Essential Oils on Biofrequency

Aroma Chemistry

Therapeutic Effect of Various Essential Oils components

Volatility of Essential oils

Extraction Methods

Quality Control Of Essential Oils

Concepts of Purity

Plant Families

Profile Of Important Essential Oils.

Profile of other Important essential oils.

Carriers and Carrier Oils

Compendium of Vegetable oils (Fatty Acids Chart)

Carrier Oils used in Aromatherapy.

Understanding Aromatherapy

The art of healing using plant essential oils.

'AROMA' derives from the Greek word 'Spice', today the word is used more broadly to mean Fragrance; 'THERAPY' means curative treatment by the use of aromatic essential oils. Though the name is a misnomer giving an impression that the therapy works only by smelling, actually it consists of the use of aromatic essences or oils extracted from wild or cultivated plants for therapeutic purpose.

Aromatherapy is a form medicine, like aromatherapy draws on the plant world. Herein, whole or part of the essential oils. In Indian is known as the universe, one of his Vaidya -the healer. He forms of medicine- the as Churan (powder mix, medicine in liquid form tisanes etc.) and form (plant essential volatile and start exposed to air). It is the

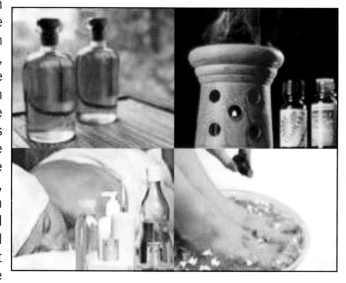

of complementary herbalism or ayurveda, the healing powers of instead of using the plant, it employs only its mythology, Lord Vishnu sustainer of the forms is the supreme has propagated three medicine in solid form Vatis/ Tablets), (herbal extracts/ medicine in gaseous oils which are highly evaporating when medicine in gaseous

form which forms the basis of today's aromatherapy. In ayurvedic practices, the essential oils are most potent of the three kind of medication used and mostly administered for treating the severe and chronic health conditions.

Plant essential oils are complex synergistic mix of various organic chemicals having varied therapeutic effect. This makes an essential oil or a combination of essential oils quite versatile in their therapeutic effect, working on us at physical, physiological and psychological level. Aromatherapy can be used at two levels –esthetic or medical. Esthetically it can be used for Skin, hair and beauty care besides massages, daily wellbeing, natural fragrance and environmental cleansing and disinfecting. Clinically it can again be used to relieve physical, physiological and psychological imbalances. The advantage is, it can be used in conjunction with traditional medicine and all other therapeutic practices or healing work, that is why it is termed as a complementary therapy.

History & Origin of Aromatherapy

The use of plants to cure diseases is as old as the human race, perhaps even older. Animals, for instance, have always sought out particular herbs or grasses when they are unwell. Man has always been dependent on the nutritional and therapeutic value of the plant world. Aromatic substances also played important roles in the medicinal practices of the Hebrew, Arabic and Indian civilizations. In the Indian mythological Epic of Ramayana, an herb called "Sanjeevani booti" had been administered by crushing, the aroma thus released, from the herb, was made to be inhaled to Laxman, the younger brother of Lord Ram, so as to revive him from unconsciousness suffered during the epic battle. Ancient Indian healing science of ayurveda had also been using plant essential oils, the difference is that aromatherapy focuses on the use of essential oils only, while in ayurveda other parts of the plant are also used.

Ancient Egyptians also used aromatherapy, as a way of life. At about the same time when the Chinese were developing acupuncture, the Egyptians were using aromatic oils and balsamic substances, in both religious rituals and medicine. Records dating back to 4500 B.C. tell of perfumed oils, scented barks and resins, of spices, aromatic vinegars, wines and beers all used in medicine, ritual, astrology and embalming. The famous Egyptian art of embalming has reflections of today's aromatherapy principles. The embalmers knew of the natural antiseptic and antibiotic properties of the plant and how these could be utilized in the process of preserving human bodies. Traces of resins like Galbanum, Frankincense, and Myrrh along with spices like Clove, Cinnamon and Nutmeg have been isolated from the bandages of the mummies. When Tutankhamen's tomb was opened in 1922, many pots were found containing substances such as Myrrh and Frankincense (both derived from tree resins), these were used for medicine as well as for perfume making, the two being interchangeable at that time.

Translations of hieroglyphics inscribed on Papyri and Stele, found in the temple of Edfu, indicate that the aromatic substances were blended to specific formulations by the high priests and alchemists to make perfumes and medicinal potions. The priests knew of the power of certain smells to raise the spirits or to promote the state of tranquility. A favorite perfume that time was Kyphi, a mixture of sixteen different essences - including myrrh and juniper - and this was inhaled to heighten the senses and spiritual awareness of the priests. The incenses, used in the present religious rituals, serve much of the same purpose.

While, the Egyptians perfected the art of using the essences of plants to control emotion, putrefaction and disease, new discoveries regarding the medicinal power of plants were continued to be made. The Greeks developed medicine from part superstition to science. Hippocrates, popularly known as the father of modem medicine, was the first physician to base medical knowledge and treatment on accurate observation, one of his beliefs was that a daily aromatic bath and scented massage were a way to health, very much the central principle of today's aromatherapy. He was aware of the anti-bacterial properties of certain plants and when an epidemic of plague broke out in Athens he urged the people to burn aromatic plants at the corners of the street to protect themselves and prevent the plague from spreading.

This was the time, when botanical knowledge was expanding, reaching its peak in the Historia plantarum of Theophrastus, the so called father of Botany. At this time there were 'immigrant' Greek physicians and seeker of knowledge who dominated the medical world. One of these was Dioscorides, a Greek surgeon in Nero's army, who wrote 'De Materia Medica' one of the most comprehensive textbook on the properties and uses of medicinal plants. It was he who recorded finer details, such as when a plant and its active principles might be at the most powerful. This indisputable fact of plant life, depending on time of day, time of the year and state of development - is utilized by the essential oil industry today. For instance, the poppy's yield in the morning is four times greater than in the evening. Jasmine's perfume and therefore its oil's aroma is strongest in the evening; this is why, jasmine flowers are still picked at night, in India, for their aromatic properties.

The Romans, were more interested in the culinary than the medical properties of the plants,they had enormous influence in the field of botany. Many herbal plants like parsley, fennel and lovage etc were introduced, in England, by Romans. The middle ages in Europe roughly from the sixth century to the Renaissance in the Fourteenth Century, was not an inspired period in terms of medical advancements. The Sixteenth and Seventeenth Centuries were the times of the great herbals in Europe. The knowledge grew in leaps and bounds, with the founding of Royal Society in Britain, the plant classification of Linnaeus, the explorations of Thomas Cook etc. Alongside there was growth of the scientific approach to medicine, though the belief in therapeutic principles of essential oils still co-existed and by the end of the eighteen century, essential oils were widely used in medicine. Once Chemistry began to flourish as a discipline and plant medicine could be synthesized in the laboratory, providing cures that were stronger and faster in action; aromatherapy and its oils began to lose their place in pharmacopeia.

Aromatherapy in the Twentieth Century

Dr. Rene Maurice Gattefosse, a French perfumery scientist is credited for the reincarnation of aromatherapy, as a form of medicine and coined the term "Aromatherapie", when he published his book by the same name in 1928, to describe the therapeutic action of aromatic plant essences. He explained in detail the properties of essential oils and their methods of application, with examples of their antiseptic, bactericidal, anti viral and anti-inflammatory properties. He described how after burning his hand in the laboratory, he plunged the hand into the nearest container, which happened to contain essential oil of Lavender and was astonished to see, how quickly the pain ceased and the skin healed. He solicited support of Dr. Jean Valnet, a medical doctor and continued to experiment with essential oils, using men in the military hospital, as his subjects during the First World War, mainly using essential oils such as Thyme, Clove, Chamomile and Lemon with astounding results. Later the work was carried on by Dr. Valnet, who had to resort to the use of essential oils, due to shortage of antibiotics during Second world war. Dr. Valnet was a holder of the Legion d'Honner and founded the Societie Francaise de Phytotherapie de l' Aromatherapie, was the president of the same and published a book called "The Practice of Aromatherapy".

Until the Second World War, essential oils of Cinnamon, Clove, Lemon, Thyme and Chamomile were used as natural disinfectants and antiseptics, to fumigate hospital wards and sterilize instruments, used in surgery and dentistry. The present usage of essential oils with carrier or base oils, involving mainly cold pressed vegetable oils, had been introduced by French biochemist Marguerite Maurey, married to an Austrian homeopath. She did extensive study on the absorption of essential oils through the skin and recommended the use of vegetable oils as the carriers in aromatherapy. She extended the scope of her work bringing aromatherapy into the world of esthetics and cosmetology, allying medicine, health and beauty.

Aromatherapy Today

Aromatherapy is now widely practiced and accepted in America, Europe, Britain and many other countries along with other alternative or better called complementary systems of healing and referred as "Medicine Douce" (Soft Medicine) in France. Due to the side effects of the synthetic drugs, people all over the world are now turning once again, to natural remedies and healing practices. Using a synthetic drug to kill harmful bacteria is like cracking a nut with a sledge hammer; not only do those kill the harmful bacteria, they also destroy the beneficial ones, present in the body. Natural remedies like essential oils, on the other hand may act slowly in antibiotic sense, but while killing off the bacteria or virus, they raise the body's immune system to strengthen its resistance to further attack, besides helping the system to rejuvenate itself, which eventually is one of its most positive effect of essential oils. The beneficial effect, the oils can have on the mind, give an added dimension to their use in healing.

All essential oils help to balance emotions to some degree and individually they may be noted for their stimulating, uplifting relaxing or euphoric properties. At psychological level, they can revive a tired mind and stimulate the memory. Interestingly, the area of the brain associated with smell is also that in which the memory is stored and aromas have been effectively used to stimulate the mind of those suffering from amnesia. Essential oils also increase our finest vibrations and assist the subtle body. They can stimulate and assist in the process of awakening, healing and opening the chakra and strengthening the aura. To understand that aspect of essential oils we have to incorporate another dimension from ayurvedic and tantric view point, analysing elements and gunas associated with them.

Observations of the effectiveness of essential oils are gradually being backed by studies taking place in parts of Central Europe, the USA, Australia and the UK. All essential oils appear to be antiseptic and bactericidal to some degree and some may also be helpful in the treatment of viral infections which are resistant to all known orthodox medicines. Many essential oils have the potential to stimulate healthy cell renewal and growth, and to regulate and restore balance of the mind and body systems. Essential oils are noted too, for their ability to reduce stress and stimulate sluggish circulation. These qualities, combined with their regenerative powers, give strength to their claims that they boost the immune system.

With the renewed interest towards natural and complementary therapies essential oils offer a new approach to holistic health and healing beyond beauty and spa treatments, specially, as a way to good health or rehabilitation therapy.

Nature of Essential oils

Essential oils are the odoriferous liquid components of plants, trees and grasses. They influence growth and reproduction, attract pollinating insects, repel predators and protect the plant from disease. Unlike 'fixed' or fatty oils, they are highly volatile, which means they evaporate if left in the open air. Many essences have the consistency of water or alcohol such as lavender, chamomile and rosemary. Others, such as Myrrh and Vertivert are viscous or thick and sticky, whereas the exquisite Rose otto is semi-solid at room temperature but becomes liquid with the slightest warmth.

The essential oils are stored in tiny oil glands or sacs which are concentrated in different parts of the plant. They may be found in the petals (Rose), leaves (Eucalyptus), roots of grass (Vertivert), heart wood (Sandalwood), rind of the fruit (Lemon), seeds (Caraway), rhizomes (Ginger) or resin (Pine) and sometimes in more than one part of the plant. Lavender, for instance yields oil from both the flowers and the leaves, while the orange tree produces three different smelling essences with varying therapeutic properties; the heady bitter-sweet Neroli (flower blossom) and a similar though less refined essence of Petit grain (leaves) and the cheery Orange (rind/skin of the fruit). The more oil glands present in the plant, the cheaper the oil, and vice versa. For instance 100 kilos of Lavender yields almost 3 liters of essential oil, whereas 1000 kilos of Rose petals can yield only half a liter.

Each essential oil is a complex synergistic mix of a range of various organic chemicals and a dynamic concentrated representation of the healing properties of the plant. It is believed to contain its life force, having certain therapeutic or balancing effect. Because of this synergy they do not disturb body's natural balance or homeostasis; if one component has a strong effect another component acts as a balancer or quencher, therefore making essential oils highly versatile and safe in healing practice. Essential oils are highly concentrated substances and rarely used neat, though neat Lavender essence is sometimes used in aromatherapy as a first aid and as an antiseptic.

In aromatherapy, inhalation, application and baths are the principle methods used to encourage essential oils to enter the body. Since essential oils are highly volatile, evaporating readily on exposure to air, and when inhaled may enter the body via the olfactory system, when diluted and applied externally, essential oil molecules may permeate skin. Bath treatments enable you to both inhale and absorb the oils. Once within your system, essential oils will work to re-establish harmony and revitalize those systems or organs where there is a malfunction or lack of balance. Their effects are many and varied, but they are noted for their antiseptic properties and their ability to restore balance to both body & mind.

Essential oils also act on the central nervous system- some will relax (Chamomile, Lavender, Rose otto); others will stimulate (Rosemary, Jasmine, Black pepper, Eucalyptus). A few have the ability to 'normalize', for example Hyssop can raise low blood pressure and lower high blood pressure. Likewise, Bergamot and Geranium can either sedate or stimulate according to individual needs. Some researchers have indicated that essential oils like holy Basil can increase atmospheric oxygen and provide negative ions, inhibiting bacterial growth thereby rendering them as antibacterial and anti infectious.

How Essential Oils Work

Essential oils are used as a gentle approach to healthcare, to aid skincare, soothe and promote relaxation and simply to seduce us with the world of fragrant treasures. These oils work on us at physical, physiological and psychological level. At psychological level they work through inhalation while skin application helps at physical and physiological level. Another benefit of essential oils is at the subtle level for cleansing aura and chakras, besides cleansing the environment from negative energies; that had been the reason for their use in all spiritual practices.

PSYCHOLOGICAL EFFECT-

The part of the brain, which identifies aromas, is called the limbic section or the central part of the brain; it's also responsible for our memory and emotions. When inhaled, essential oils molecules are taken directly to the olfactory system, which actually is a patch of cells located at the roof our nose. This patch of cells have a thin hair like protruding called cilia, which registers and transmits information about the aromas to our brain via the olfactory nerve which is directly connected to the brain. When electro-chemical messages are forwarded to this limbic section of brain about the smell, it triggers the release of neuro-chemicals, which may result in relaxing, uplifting, sedative or euphoric effect on our body through our pituitary gland. The balancing effect the essential oils can have on the mind, lends an added dimension to their use in healing stress related / psycho somatic disorders. All essential oils help to balance emotions to some degree and individually they may be noted for their specific effect like relaxing, uplifting, sedative, euphoric; they can revive a tired mind stimulate memory and emotions.

Process of olfaction-

When inhaled, essential oil molecules, in vapor form, travel directly to the roof of the nose to the olfactory cells. The cilia from each receptor cell registers and transmits information about the quality of aroma to the brain through electrochemical messages, which are processed in the limbic section and a neuro chemical message transmitted to pituitary which in turn releases various hormones leading to the physical effect.

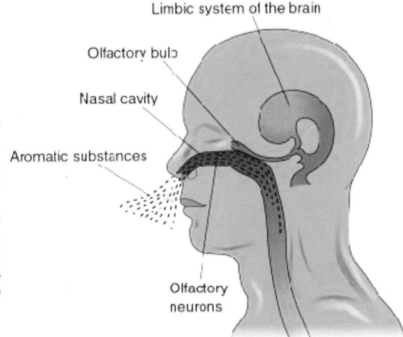

Limbic system of the brain

Olfactory bulb

Nasal cavity

Aromatic substances

Olfactory neurons

PHYSICAL / PHYSIOLOGICAL EFFECT

When dissolved in a carrier oil and rubbed into the skin or when dispersed in water used for bath, tiny essential oils molecules, being volatile in nature, readily permeate the skin via the skin pores and hair follicles.

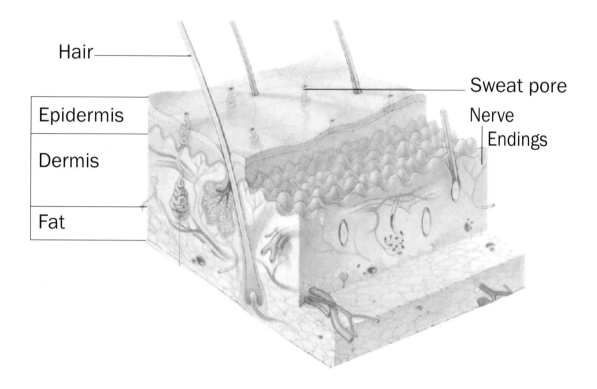

Hair

Sweat pore

Epidermis

Nerve
Endings

Dermis

Fat

They reach the body's circulatory system through the lymphatic vessels. Once in the blood stream they are transported around the body and filtered through to the body fluids passing their therapeutic benefits to the entire body. Since essential oils with inherent therapeutic properties are able to keep infection at bay, they in fact boost the entire functioning of the immune system.

Effect of Essential Oils on Biofrequency

For years, research has been conducted on the use of electrical energy to reverse disease. Scientists in the field of natural and energy healing have believed there has to be more natural way to increase the body's electrical frequency. This led to the research and subsequent discovery of electrical frequencies in essential oils.

Every living thing has energy which can be measured in terms of electrical frequency because frequency is a measurable rate of electrical energy that is constant between any two points. Considerable research has been done; Robert O. Becker, MD documented the electrical frequency of the human body in his book called *"The Body Electric"*. Bruce Tainio of Tainio Technology in Cheney, Washington developed an equipment to measure the biofrequency of humans and foods, he used biofrequency monitors to determine and disease. Measuring in megahertz typically has a frequency ranging from disease sets in at 58 MHZ. This energy negative thought. In studies it was lowered the measured frequency of a thoughts raised the measured that prayer and meditation increased Mhz. This gives credence to the fact anxiety, depression etc. do result in

> It was found that a healthy body typically has a frequency ranging from 62 to 78 MHz. while the process of disease sets in at 58 MHZ

the relationship between frequency (MHz), it was found that a healthy body 62 to 78 MHz. while the process of level gets disturbed even by a single observed that negative thoughts person upto 12 MHz and positive frequency by 10 Mhz. It was also found the measured frequency levels by 15 that prolonged levels of Stress, lowering the body energy as well as immune levels, allowing the disease to set in, as the case is in all psycho somatic disorders.

It was also observed in those studies that processed / canned food had a zero to minimal MHz frequency, fresh produce dry herbs from 12- 22 MHz, 20-27 Mhz. Essential oils highest frequency of natural MHz and went as high as frequency of Rose Oil. In this frequencies of essential oils

> Essential oils are found to have the highest frequency of natural substance, starting at 52 MHz and went as high as 320 MHz, that's the frequency of Rose Oil.

measured up to 15 Mhz, while the fresh herbs from are found to have the substance, starting at 52 320 MHz, that's the sense, the chemistry and have the ability to help man maintain optimal health frequency, providing an environment where microbes cannot live.

When essential oils are diffused it was observed that patients felt better emotionally, within seconds of exposure to the oils and inhalation of the same, felt calm and less anxious. It is fascinating to see the way the oils work on the body, certain oils acted within seconds while others acted in 1-3 minutes, when the oil applied on the feet could travel to the head and take effect within a minute. The more the results people got, more and more studies are being initiated, in this field.

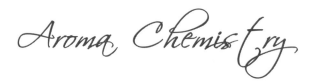

Aroma Chemistry

The primary and secondary metabolism of the plants had been a subject of study for organic and bio chemists. The way plants make essential oils gives some insight into their complexity. The chemical components of an essential oil are produced during second stage of biosynthesis and thus secondary metabolites.

A distilled essential oil is a mixture of various organic chemicals, some of them were present as natural constituents of the oil, at the time of distillations, others are formed during processing by the hydrolysis of glycosides, while a few are formed by partial decomposition of delicate natural components.

The chemistry of essential oils is complex and the components of the essential oils can broadly be classified as terpenes, esters, aldehydes, ketones, alcohols, phenols and oxides. Since essential oils are composed of a wide range of different chemicals, they will have different therapeutic effects and exert different effects on the body. This explains why a single essential oil has a wide range of therapeutic properties, Lavender for example, balances the central nervous system, and it is also a wonderful skin healing agent for problems such as athlete's foot, bed sores, acne and eczema. The essential oil can also be used in the bath or blended into a massage oil, for relaxation or therapeutic massage to relieve conditions like muscular pain and rheumatism, and much more. It is also interesting to note that resins such as frankincense & myrrh containing resin alcohols have a similar chemical structure to human steroids (the male and female hormones). Whether resins alcohols exert a hormone stimulating effect on human has not been officially proven, in the affirmative. Of course, much more research into this area is needed before we can jump to any firm conclusions.

The gas chromatograph can separate out the main components of essential oils by looking at the 'chemical fingerprint' produced. However, the pattern of the living essence is complex beyond the chemist's ability to replicate the exact aroma by mixing together the various chemical components. Something is always missing in the 'nature identical' version. Following are the main components and therapeutic effects of the various isolated constituents found in essential oils.

Terpenes: Terpenes make up the largest single group of compounds in essential oils. Normally their name end in "ene", terpenes are made up of a chain, of 5 carbon atoms, one of them having a double bond, known as an isoprene unit. Depending on the number of isoprene units in a terpenic compound, it can be classified as Mono, sesqui or Di terpene.

Monoterpene- is composed of two isoprene units. It is the basic terpene unit and make up the largest group of terpenes. They are light molecules hence evaporate quickly when exposed to air, thus represent themselves in top note. Since isoprene units making the terpene have double bonds, hence terpense are prone to oxidation therefore they are photosensitive. That is why essential oils rich in terpene have shorter shelf life.

Common terpenes include limonene (an antiviral agent found in 90 per cent of citrus oils), pinene (an antiseptic found in high concentrations in pine and terpentine oils), camphene and myrcene. They are light antiseptic and have uplifting and stimulating effect on the nervous system.

Sesquiterpenes are composed of three isoprene units, making them slightly heavier and less volatile. They have stronger odor, have anti inflammatory and bactericidal properties; common examples are chamazulene (German Chamomile), bisabolene (black pepper), and caryophyllene (ylang ylang).

Di terpenes are heavy molecules made up of four isoprene units, not common as they tend to react with hydroxyl groups to form terpinic alcohols. This process in Clary sage produces sclareol, a component known for its hormone balancing effect.

Alcohols: Terpinic alcohols, ending in "ol" are found in many essential oils. They are the result of the reaction of terpenes with hydroxyl groups (oh). Monoterpinic alcohols are good antisepticswith some antibacterial and antifungal properties. Some alcohols are uplifting, others like linalool have sedative effect, while isoborneol inhibits herpes virus (Armaka et al 1999). Di terpenic alcohols like sclareol have hormone regulating effect.

Essential oils having a higher percentage of monoterpinic alcohols are safe to be used on skin, even undiluted. Some of the most common terpenic alcohols include linalol (found in lavender), citronellol (rose and geranium) and geraniol (geranium and palmarosa). These substances tend to give good antiseptic, antiviral properties and uplifting qualities to essential oils.

Esters: The most widespread group found in plant essences ending in "ate"; esters are combination of an acid with an alcohol, like linalylic acid and alcohol produce linalyl acetate found in Clary sage and Lavender, geranyl acetate is found in Geranium and sweet marjoram. Esters are fungicidal, antispasmodic and sedative, usually with a fruity aroma.

Aldehydes: These substances are found notably in lemon scented essences, ending in "al" like citral in Lemongrass and Citronella, Cinnamic aldehyde in Cinnamon oil, are strong chemicals which can sensitize the skin should therefore be used with caution. Aldehydes generally have anti depressant and uplifting quality.

Ketones: The ketones found in pennyroyal, tansy, sage and wormwood are actually toxic, which is why these essences are best avoided by the layperson. Ending in "one" they are aromatic chemicals with strong aroma. However, not all ketones are dangerous. Non-toxic ketones include jasmone, found in Jasmine, and fenchone in Sweet Fennel. Ketone eases congestion and aides the flow of mucus, which is why plants and essences containing these substances are helpful for upper respiratory complaints.

Phenols: These are bactericidal with a strong & stimulating effect on the central nervous system. They are aromatic group alcohols, also end in "ol" However, they are stronger chemicals and can also be skin irritants, especially if isolated from the whole essential oil and used as single 'active principle'. Common phenols are eugenol in Clove oil and thymol in Thyme oil, are potentially harmful, it is best to avoid using these essences, at least for skin use. Clove essence, for instance, can be safely used in room perfumes.

Oxides- These are found in a wide range of essences, especially those of camphoraceous nature such as eucalyptus oil which contains an oxide called 1-8 cineol or eucalyptol, having an expectorant effect.

Lectones- Lectones are present in all expressed oils, the percentage may be low but they play an important role as expectorant and mucolytic, although some lactones have neurotoxic effect as ketones.

Coumarins- Coumarins are a type or sub group like lactones. They may be present in an oil, in smaller quantity and have antispasmodic effect. A certain group of coumarins present in citrus peels like bergaptine in Bergamot, also found in Angelica root is found to react in the presence of ultraviolet light, can cause photo toxicity.

Ethers- Ethers are responsible for some of the hallucinogenic properties of certain essential oils when taken orally.

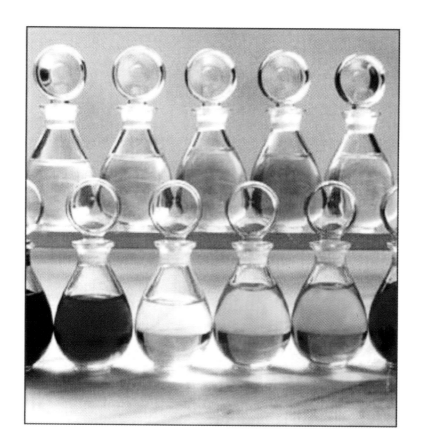

Therapeutic Effect of various essential oil's components

By knowing active ingredients responsible for certain therapeutic effect you can choose the best oils for your needs.

	ACIDS	ALCOHOLS (MONO)	ALCOHOLS (SESQUI)	ALDEHYDES	COUMARINS	ESTERS	ETHERS (PHENOLIC)	KETONES	LACTONES	OXIDES	PHENOLS	TERPENES (MONO)	TERPENES (SESQUI)
ABORTIFACIENT								X					
ANALGESIC								X			X	X	X
AIR ANTISEPTIC											X		
ANTI-SEPTIC				X							X		X
ANTI-COAGULANT					X			X					
ANTI-FUNGAL		X		X		X		X					
ANTI-INFECTIOUS		X		X			X				X		
ANTI-INFLAMMATORY	X			X		X	X	X					X
ANTI-SPASMODIC						X	X				X		X
ANTI-VIRAL		X		X							X	X	
BACTERICIDAL		X									X	X	X
BALANCING						X							
CICATRISANT						X		X			X		
DECONGESTANT (circulatory)			X										
DIGESTIVE								X			X		
DIURETIC											X		
EXPERCTORANT								X		X	X	X	
HEPATIC		X	X										
HYPOTENSIVE			X	X	X								X
IMMUNE SYSTEM BALANCER		X											
IMMUNO STIMULANT											X		
LIPOLYTIC								X					
MUCOLYTIC								X	X	X	X		
NEUROTOXIC								X					
PHOTOTOXIC					X								
RELAXANT					X	X	X	X				X	
SEDATIVE						X	X	X			X		
SKIN IRRITANT				X							X	X	X
SKIN SENSITIZING				X					X				
STIMULANT	X							X				X	
TEMPERATURE REDUCING			X	X						X			
TONIC, NERVE (UPLIFTING)	X	X			X	X	X				X		
TONIC (GENERAL)	X	X			X								
VASOCONSTRICTIVE	X												
WARMING	X										X		

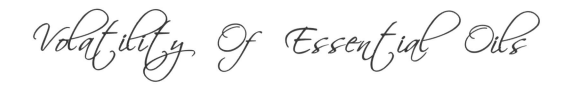

Volatility Of Essential Oils

Volatility of essential oils is the rate of evaporation of its components.

You can smell the aroma of certain essential oils as soon as you open the bottle, while in some, you need to bring a container close to your nose to get the whiff of the aroma. This is because various oils evaporate at different rate, depending upon its composition. The organic chemicals which make up an essential oil can be light or heavy. An essential oil composed of more of light chemicals, evaporate quickly and instantly hit your nose, we call them "TOP NOTE" oils. Mostly mono terpenes, mono terpenols, ketones, phenols, aldehydes, and oxides show themselves in top notes, hence oils with higher percentage of these components have strong aroma. When an oil is having mid size chemicals, comparatively slower to evaporate they show themselves in "MIDDLE NOTES" like seqsui terpenes, sesqui terpenols, esters, alcohols etc. While the heavy components, like di terpenes, di terpenols, wax esters etc take longer to evaporate they are called "BASE NOTE"; these components act as natural fixatives as they help to hold the lighter components. These base note oils are also good moisturizers as they help bind moisture to the skin.

All fragrances whether natural or synthetic can therefore be classified as top, middle and bottom notes. In a perfume or essential oil (single oil, may contain more than one note), top note is the initial aroma you get followed by middle notes, which are slightly different but longer lasting. They make up the body of the perfume and what you get to smell when the perfume has almost evaporated are the bottom or base notes.

The art of blending involves creating a balance of Top, Middle and Bottom note oils or components. Normally we use a combination of 3 to 5 essential oils, as they are synergists. Whether you are mixing oils for vaporization, bath or as a perfume besides the therapeutic effect you need to be aware of the aroma effect of the oil as the overall effect should be as desired.

AROMATHERAPY TOP NOTES- Aromas classified as top notes are highly uplifting, stimulating the mind, relieve depression. They are cleansing and invigorating, help clear congestions and colds, also help in respiratory conditions. Typical top note oils are citrus, leafy, camphoraceous or minty for example- Lemon, Lime, Bergamot, Grape fruit, Lemongrass, Melissa, Peppermint, Spearmint, Basil, Rosemary, Eucalyptus, Jasmine etc.

AROMATHERAPY MIDDLE NOTES- Most of the Middle note oils are extracted from flowers, berries, herbs, spices etc. They are mostly relaxing and healing, help reduce hypertension, also good for PMS and related symptoms. Typical examples are- Lavender, Geranium, chamomiles, Clary sage, Ylang Ylang Juniperberry, Marjoram, Clove, Nutmeg, Black Pepper, Ginger etc.

AROMATHERAPY BOTTOM/ BASE NOTES - Base note oils are soothing, relaxing, sedatives, lingering and help restore emotional balance. Most of the oils extracted from roots, wood, stems, bark and resins, they are used as fixatives and moisturizers. Typical examples are- Vertiver, Patchauli, Sandalwood, Cedarwood, Myrrh, Benzoin, Jatamansi, Valerian root oil etc.

Extraction Methods

Essential oils are contained in the glands, veins, sacs and glandular hairs of aromatic plants. Flowers, leaves and non-fibrous parts need little, if any, preparation prior to distillation. Tough stalks, woody parts, roots, seeds and fruits, however, need to be 'comminuted' (cut up, disintegrated or crushed-wood is grated) in order to rupture the cell walls, allowing the easy escape of the volatile oil.

The basic principles for extracting essential oils from plants remain the same as of hundreds of years ago, though tremendous advances have been made in the techniques used and the methods employed. The oil extractors objective is to extract essential oil in the most natural form. Distillation is and no doubt will continue to be, the most preferred extraction method.

During distillation, only very tiny molecules can evaporate, so they are the only ones which leave the plant. These extremely small molecules make up an essential oil. Oils containing more of the smallest molecules are most volatile and termed 'top notes' in the perfumery world; those containing more of the heaviest and least volatile of tiny molecules are called 'base notes'. Those in between are known as middle or sometimes 'heart' or 'middle' notes.

Steam Distillation-

Distillation is still considered, to be, one of the most economical method, of extracting essential oils from plant materials. Some plants have to be distilled immediately after they are harvested, for example Melissa, if left, even for a few hours, the essential oil is lost; hence the yield from Melissa is, in any case, very low. Some plants are left a few days, e.g. Lavender, so that surplus water in the plant can dry out this by the way, slightly affects the yield. Some, like Black Pepper seeds, Clary sage and

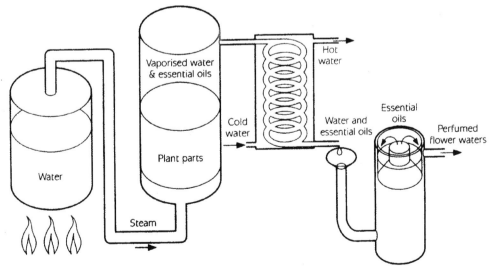

Steam Distillation Process

Peppermint, can be totally dried before distilling without losing any essential oil. There is an art of distillation and that, especially for low-yield plants, much skill is needed. The aim of the distiller is to achieve an oil, as close as possible, the way oil exists in the plant.

When plant parts are heated by steam in still, the essential oils present in the plant material are freed, evaporating into the steam. These tiny molecules are carried along in a pipe together with the steam and as they get further away from the heat source they begin to cool. To hasten this process, the pipe passes through a large vat of cold water, called condenser, where steam condenses back into liquid form. As the density of essential oil differs from that of water, it either floats on the top or sinks to the bottom (mostly the former) where it can be drawn off. The result is pure, genuine, whole and natural essential oil- an Aromatherapist's dream

Carbon Dioxide Extraction -

This is a fairly new method of extracting essential oils, introduced at the beginning of the 1980s, utilizing compressed carbon dioxide. The technology calls for an expensive and complicated equipment, which utilizes carbon dioxide at very high pressures and extremely low temperature. With this method, more top notes, fewer terpenes, a higher proportion of esters, plus larger molecules can also be obtained. The resultant oil is said to be better and more like the essential oil in the plant, in a distilled oil many terpenes seem to form during the distillation process, which also breaks down some of the acetates (esters) in the plant material.

Carbon dioxide(CO_2) extracted essential oils are pure and stable, colorless and have no residue of CO_2 left in them- thus they are excellent therapeutically, although this needs to be verified for each oil on account of their different compositions.

This method is not suitable for all oils, there are still a few practical difficulties to overcome (sometimes an emulsion is produced).

Hydro- diffusion or Percolaction-

Percolation is more recent than CO, extraction. It is an extremely interesting process, as most of the resultant oils had an aroma nearer to the plant, better than a distilled oil. The equipment, unlike that for CO_2 extraction, is very simple and the process quicker than distillation, the plant being in contact with the steam for a much shorter time, thus truer to nature.

This process works like a coffee percolator. The steam passes through the plant material from top to bottom of the container, which has a grid to hold the plant material. The oil and condensed steam is collected in a vessel in the same way as distillation. The color of oils thus is much richer than that of distilled oils as time and tests alone will reveal their true value in aromatherapy.

Expression-
This method of extraction is used exclusively with citrus fruits, where the essential oil, located in little sacs just under the surface of the rind, simply needs to be pressed out.

Expression is usually carried out by a factory producing fruit juice, thus maximizing the profit from the whole fruit. Expressed oil is taken directly from the fresh peel without heat, it is recommended that citrus oils for therapeutic use, be obtained from organically or naturally grown produce.

Cold-pressed citrus oils are special, in that they are known to be exactly of the same composition as in the plant itself, hence preferred. In many juice/essential oil factories the peel is steam distilled after expression, which releases even more oil (though of a poorer quality).

In the past, the oil was extracted by hand (and collected in sponges), the size of the industry today necessitates expression by machinery and the process is known as 'sacrification'. With expression, both volatile and large molecules, such as waxes and other substances, are contained in the finished product, while by distillation only tiny molecules can be collected.

The shelf life of expressed oils is shorter than that of distilled oils, they are recommended to be stored in a cool, dark place (many people choose the refrigerator).

Solvent Extraction-

Absolutes and resinoids are obtained by solvent extraction and not classed as essential oils. They are highly concentrated perfume materials, containing those plant molecules which are soluble in the solvents, used to extract them.

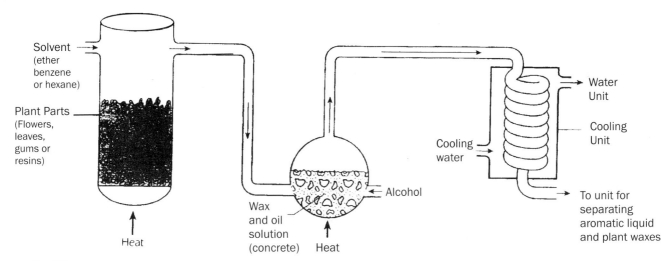

Resinoids:

Resins are the solid or semi-solid substances exuded from the bark of trees or bushes when wounded (cut, as in a rubber tree). The gum-like substance produced does not exist in the tree before and but is produced pathologically, solely as a result of the incision, and hardens on exposure to air. Various solvents can be used to extract the aromatic molecules from the resin, the most frequently used being hydrocarbons (e.g. benzene, hexane) or alcohols-each extracting different molecules. The solvents are filtered off and afterward removed by distillation to leave either resinoids (from hydrocarbon solvents) or absolute resins (from alcohol solvents). Commonly used absolutes from resins and their extracts in aromatherapy are Frankincense, Benzoin, Myrrh, Elmi and Galbanum.

Concretes:

The extraction of concretes is similar to that of resinoids (hydrocarbons are used as solvents). For concretes however, plant material (leaves, flowers roots, etc.) is used instead of a resins this is the main difference. Most concretes are solid, wax-like substances and are much used in food flavorings.

Absolutes:

An absolute is prepared from a concrete, by adding an alcohol to extract the aromatic (alcohol-soluble) molecules. The alcohol is then evaporated off gently under vaccum, leaving the absolute, a thick, colored liquid. The total process is much more complicated.

Absolutes and resins always retain a small percentage of the solvents used in their production, hence not preferred for aromatherapy work, but they are much used in the perfumery world. Some solvents may cause substance sensitivity on certain skins, depending on the quality and quantity of the retained solvent. Jasmine absolute, a favorite aroma for many people and possibly the most important fragrance to the perfume industry (there is no essential oil of jasmine available), is extremely vulnerable to adulteration and available at a wide range of prices (reflecting the quality).

Enfleurage:

Pomades were obtained from the enfleurage process used long ago (replaced by concretes), when petals or leaves were laid on trays of animal fat for many days, being replaced regularly until the fat used as a solvent was saturated with the plant extracts.

Quality Control of Essential Oils

In practice of aromatherapy, quality of essential oils play a very important role, when people are trying to cash on the popularity of aromatherapy by dishing out all sorts of essential oils from synthetic/ reconstituted or nature identical to adulterated. So, we have to be cautious of the quality of essential oils we use for therapy purpose else the desired result will not come.

Traditionally, the purpose of quality control has always been to make sure that substandard products do not reach the customer. It is very important to check the quality of essential oils, since optimum quality is paramount not only in order to get best results but also to avoid possible harmful side effects. Another bonus is that less essential oil is thus needed in order to be effective, a fact people overlook while buying cheap oils, on pretext of false economy of price.

The essential oils quality can be tested by Non-analytical physical tests or Analytical tests.

NON-ANALYTICAL PHYSICAL TESTS

Non-analytical physical tests give information on certain properties of essential oils, though not on their composition-

Appearance- The appearance of an essential oil is no criterion of good quality, but may forewarn of poor quality. Most distilled oils, of high quality, are transparent or slightly hazy; a definitely hazy or cloudy, essential oil is always of questionable quality. Absolutes frequently present a hazy, translucent or even opaque appearance. Expressed citrus oils are always colored and show natural color variations due to difference in the pigmentation in the outer rind of the fruit.

Viscosity - The term viscosity is used to refer to the thickness of a liquid or, more scientifically, to its resistance to flow, commonly seen in high viscosity liquids such as glycerin. Water, conversely, is a mobile liquid, one of low viscosity. All expressed and mostly distilled oils used in aromatherapy are mobile liquids; while a few like Sandalwood, Vertiver, Jatamansi are viscous. Few essential oils, like Orris oil, for example are solid at room temperature.

Specific Gravity- The specific gravity of a solid or liquid is a measure of how much heavier or lighter a given volume of the substance is than the same volume of pure water, measured at a standard temperature. Measurement of specific gravity are usually made at $20^{\circ}C$. Most essential oils are lighter than water and have values of specific gravity less than 1, but a few, for example clove oil, are heavier and collect beneath the distillation water during extraction.

Specific gravity now is measured by means of an electronic specific gravity meter which gives the result and temperature of the sample on a small LCD display screen.

Refractive Index- When you lower a needle into a bowl of water at an angle of about 60° to the horizontal, the needle appears to bend towards the surface as it enters the water and to unbend as it is withdrawn. This optical effect is called refraction, caused by the reduction of speed of light when passing from a less dense medium (in this case air) into a denser medium (water). The refraction of a ray of light passing from air into a transparent liquid or solid medium is expressed numerically as the refractive index of the denser medium with respect to the air, for example an essential oil.

As in case of specific gravity, a specification of refractive index is expressed as upper and lower limits between which, at the given temperature, the refractive index of the test sample should lie.

The property of the refraction of light by a substance can be very responsive to small changes of composition, and so in respect of an essential oil a value for refractive index which is greater or lesser than the limits of the specified range is regarded as an early warning of the possibility of poor quality, to the extent of adulteration.

Refractive index is measured by means of a refractometer, using a thin film of test sample mounted on a temperature controlled stage, similar to the stage of a microscope. A standard light source gives a visual field, viewed through one of the two eyepieces, consisting of adjacent semicircles of colored light. The field is adjusted by the operator to show an even distribution of color, whereupon the refractive index of the sample is obtained on a scale, visible through the other eye piece. Electronic refracto meters give direct readings of refractive index, free from human observational error.

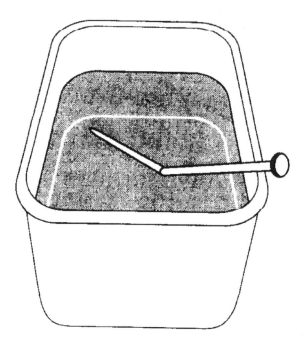

Refraction of light
using knitting needle in water

Examples of refractive indices of essential oils are as follows:

Bergamot Oil	1.464 to 1.467
Clove Bud Oil	1.528 to 1.537
Lavender Oi	1.459 to 1.464
Lemongrass Oil	1.483 to 1.489
Rosemary Oil	1.464 to 1.476
Sandalwood Oil	1.500 to 1.510

Optical Rotation- Light waves are analogous to the waves produced in a long length of rope, secured at one end, when the opposite end is moved energetically up and down; they are traverse waves, propagated in a plane perpendicular to the surface to which rope is secured. A filter of a different kind, given by polarized lens of the kind used for sunglasses is used to measure optical rotation of essential oils. Since this material absorbs all rays of light passing through it excepting those traveling in a particular plane called the plane of polarization. Rays emerging from such a filter are plane polarized, meaning that all of them travel in a parallel planes.

To measure optical rotation, a horizontal glass tube, usually 10 cms in length is fitted with plane glass ends, is filled with the liquid under examination. The temperature of the tube and contents are adjusted to a level between 15 and 20° C and the tube is then placed horizontally in a polariscope, the instrument used to measure optical rotation. A beam of plane-polarised light of sodium wavelength is passed through the liquid in a polariscope tube and is viewed at the opposite end through an eyepiece fitted with a second polarizing lens secured to a circular scale marked in angular degrees. The scale is rotated until the two halves of an illuminated field, as viewed through the eyepiece, are equally illuminated, whereupon a reading is taken from the scale.

If the liquid in the polariscope tube is optically inactive like water, the scale of reading will be zero, in fact the zero reading of the instrument is checked in this way if necessary to be zeroed before a measurement is made. If the liquid is optically active, its effect on the plane- polarized light waves emerging from the first polarizing lens, the polarizer, is to twist them clockwise or anticlockwise as they pass through it. Hence to obtain a uniformly illuminated viewing field, the second polarizing lens, the analyzer, will have to be rotated by moving the circular scale to which it is attached. The angle of optical rotation is then obtained from the scale reading.

Liquids which rotate, the plane of the polarized light, to the right i.e. clockwise, are said to be dextro-rotatory, and the names of the organic compounds of this nature are prefixed as d-, for example d-limonene. Liquids which rotate the plane of polarized light to the left, i.e. anticlockwise, are laevo-rotatory, the names of laevo-rotatory compounds are prefixed l-, as in l-limonene. The explanation of optical activity throws light, so as to speak, on the composition of essential oils, since optical activity is caused by a particular feature of molecular structure in which an atom , particularly a carbon atom is bonded to four different atoms or group of atoms.

(A) Zero effect with water

(B) rotation of light passing through optically active liquid

The optical rotation of an essential oil is a summation of the optical rotations of its constituents, in relation to their proportions in the oil. Variations of these proportions therefore can give rise to variations of the optical rotation of the oil, thereby affecting the therapeutic properties of the oil. Measurement of optical rotation is an important aid to the detection of adulteration where, for example a deficiency of a major, optically active constituent has been corrected by the addition of the corresponding, non-stereo specific synthetic chemical, since the optical activity of the aroma chemical will be different than the natural component, adulteration of the oil with aroma chemical will therefore alter the value of its optical rotation.

ANALYTICAL CHEMICAL TESTS

Analytical chemistry may be defined as the science and art of determining the composition of material in terms of the elements or compounds contained.

Analytical tests are, basically, of two different kinds;

    a) **QUALITATIVE-** giving information on what is present in a substance;

    b) **QUANTITATIVE-** giving information on how much constituent of a mixture or element present in a compound.

From the results of qualitative tests on an essential oil, the identity of one or more of its different constituents may be ascertained after separation from the oil.

ACID VALUE – With advancing age contents of free acid in many essential oils tends to increase. This increase results mainly from the oxidation of aldehydes and hydrolysis of esters to form equivalent quantities of organic acids, the stronger of which can catalyze the further hydrolysis of esters.

The measurement of acid content of an essential oil, expressed as acid value, and comparison of result with the acid value quoted as the maximum acceptable in the specification for the oil, gives an indication of the condition and age of the product and by inference its likely rate of deterioration- a guide to whether the oil is usable or not. In the absence of deterioration, the proportion of free acid to be found in most essential oils is very small.

Determination of Esters- Some essential oils, Lavender, for example are valued for their content of natural esters (linalyl acetate and other esters in case of lavender), an ester value lower than the prescribed in the specification is a certain indication of poor quality.

Quantitative information on an essential oil with respect to its content of single constituents is usually obtained by the technique of Gas Liquid Chromatography. However chemical tests are also used to evaluate quality in respect of all constituents of a particular chemical class, present in an oil, for example, the total percentage of esters calculated as linalyl acetate, present in Lavender oil.

GAS LIQUID CHROMATOGAPHY- Chromatography is one of the analytical methods, which is basically a separation of components present in a chemical mixture. Chromatography may be regarded as an analytical technique employed for the purification and separation of organic and inorganic substances.

Gas Liquid Chromatography (GLC) is different than the column chromatography, and is more advanced, also called as Capillary GLC, used in perfumery and essential oils analysis for its sensitivity, separating

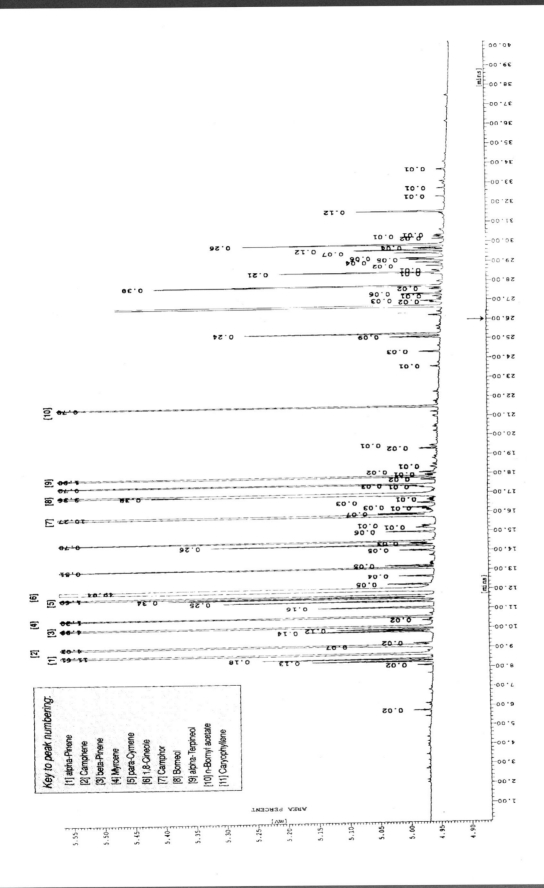

Gas Liquid Chromatograph of Rosemary Oil

Key to peak numbering:

[1] alpha-Pinene
[2] Camphene
[3] beta-Pinene
[4] Myrcene
[5] para-Cymene
[6] 1,8-Cineole
[7] Camphor
[8] Borneol
[9] alpha-Terpineol
[10] n-Bornyl acetate
[11] Caryophyllene

power and reproducibility of results. The column takes the form of a narrow silica tube of less than 1 mm internal diameter and from 30 to 100 m in length; this is wound into a coil on a former and is coated, on the inside with a very thin film of a non volatile substance. The column is secured within a temperature regulated, thermostatically controlled oven, the temperature of which can be computer programmed to increase, over a period of about 30 minutes, from room temperature to above 300° C. This is important to ensure that all constituents, from the least volatile to most volatile are vaporized slowly.

One end of the column is attached to a metal block, the injection block, having a fine hole, from which one minute drop of an essential oil is injected for analysis. The block is pre heated to ensure that the essential oil evaporates as soon as injected. At the point of evaporation, there is a connection to a cylinder of nitrogen gas, which is chemically inert and acts as a carrier, to carry the vapors of the sample through the column. The carrier gas is basically the moving phase in GLC analysis.

At the opposite end of the column is a device, called the detector which is connected to a pen recorder. The detector responds quantitatively to the presence of the truly minute amount of the vapors of the constituents separated by the column. The variations in this current, once amplified, are converted into exactly proportional movement of the pen recorder, in which the pen is arranged to draw a line on a sheet of paper moving slowly, the pen draws a peak on the paper as a permanent record of its presence and proportions in the sample. The electrical signals (changes of current) produced by the detector are fed also into a dedicated computer known as integrator, which, on completion of analysis prints out sets of figures from which the constituents of the sample can be identified and their true proportions calculated.

For the results of different GLC analyses to be comparable, the conditions of column parameters (length, diameter, composition and thickness of the stationary phase etc.) and temperature, temperature programming, nature and flow of carrier gas, all have to be standardized and kept the same from one analysis to the next.

The purpose, of the routine evaluation of fresh supply of essential oil received is to compare the chromatograph with the corresponding, standard samples which are of known composition and which conform in each case to the quality required.

Infrared Spectrophotometery (IRS)- The technique of infrared spectrophotometery involves measuring of the energy of different parts, of the spectrum of infrared radiation. Applied to an essential oil, IRS gives an overall picture, or fingerprint, of the composition of the oil. The IR spectrograph is very sensitive to small differences of composition, and so is a most useful aid to the comparison of test and standard samples of essential oils, and to the detection of adulteration. The technique has also the advantage of being able to detect and record the presence of non-volatile, as well as volatile constituents of essential oils, and of requiring only a few minutes for the completion of a spectrum.

Mass Spectrometry- This analytical technique is a powerful aid to the elucidation of the composition and structure of molecules of chemically pure organic compounds. For purpose of the elucidation of the molecular structure of constituents of essential oils, a pure constituent separated by GLC and represented by a single peak on a chromatograph, is transferred directly to a mass spectrometer.

Concepts of Purity

Today everybody claims that their oils are pure and natural, the word 'pure' is used to refer to a product which is free from any contamination or adulteration.

In case of essential oils there are two concepts of purity, which need to be ascertained, they are odor purity and chemical purity.

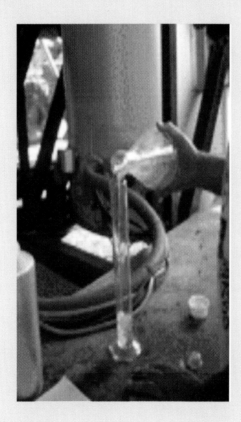

Odor Purity of an essential oil or any aromatic material may be defined as the extent to which its odor profile matches the odor profile of a standard sample of the same product and grade, when both are allowed to evaporate on smelling strips to final dry out under the same conditions at the same time. Its very important in essential oils since careful odour evaluation, at intervals during evaporation, under standard condition and comparison with standard sample, is the only test available to Aromatherapists besides visual inspection.

Chemical Purity can be checked in chemicals having identical atoms or molecules. The concept applies only to single elements or compounds. An essential oil, being a mixture of organic compounds, cannot be therefore chemically pure, even though it may be of high odor purity and 'pure 'in the sense free from contamination. The chemical composition and odor profile of an essential oil, together, provide the information, from which its purity can be ascertained, in comparison to a standard sample.

The composition and quality of essential oils is determined by the following factors –

1. **Genotype of the Plant Source** - or the genetic constitution of the plant determines the composition of the proteins forming the living matter or protoplasm, of the plant. These proteins include the enzymes which control the metabolism of the plant. In aromatic plants, essential oils are formed in oil glands or cells, their composition being determined by the enzyme controlled reaction pathways by which their constituents are synthesized.

2. **Conditions of Growth and Development of the Plant** - are very important and a major factor affecting the quality of essential oil. A green plant obtains the chemical elements that it requires

for growth and development to maturity from the surrounding atmosphere and from the soil by which it is supported. Deficiencies of any of the ions required by a plant causes poor growth and yellowing of leaves, and in aromatic plants gives poor yield of inferior quality essential oils. Atmospheric pollution can damage or destroy plant life, as can, contaminated soil.

3. **Harvesting and Processing of Aromatic Plant Material** – is another important factor, to obtain a high yield of good quality essential oil. The source material must be harvested at the time when its content of oil is at its maximum, using a technique which excludes extraneous matter, such as weed. Assuming harvesting is done properly, then another important factor to be taken care of is processing and subsequent storage of essential oil, so as to ensure completion of extraction process in the shortest possible time but under conditions of temperature and pressure that will not cause any part of the charge, in the still, to suffer damaging thermal stress.

4. **Effects of Moisture on Essential Oils** - An important factor to be taken care of, before final packing, as essential oils produced by expression or distillation frequently contain proportions of dissolved water. Some oils are comparatively more stable in presence of moisture while others like citrus plant oils are not.

5. **Storage Condition** - In general, essential oils should be stored under the following condition-

    a) In a cool place, at an even temperature,

    b) Protected from light,

    c) Under the feasible headspace of air or under nitrogen,

    d) In non plastic containers, the material of which will not in any way alter their composition.

Plant Families

The essential oils listed here are those commonly used for skin, hair and health care. When aromatherapy was first introduced, essential oils were called by their common plant name. Sometimes these single common names given to essential oils are confusing as some of the plants are unrelated, neither the same genus nor species. For example, an aromatherapist may refer to Cypress for Cupressus sempervirens, while in India; Nagarmotha is also referred and known as Cypress. The oils may contain common factors and effects are decidedly different, as in Marjorams one needs to know which essential oil from which group is needed for which purpose. In other instances the oil comes from a plant bearing the same common name and genus, but a different species, will contain a constituent not present (or present in vastly different proportion) in another similarly named genus, e.g. the eucalypti (or Eucalyptus) or garden Geranium plant, while Geranium for an aromatherapist is Pelargonium graveolens. This is confusing for a non technical person as the specific plant of a specific genus, have a different aroma as well as different therapeutic effect on human system. Therefore you need to be clear about the genus and species of the plant source.

As knowledge on the subject has deepened, the necessity of using the Latin names has become more apparent; it is now extremely important for plant oils to be identified thus. A plant may have many common names but one specific Latin name. It was Carl Linnaeus (1707 – 1778) who had established a basis of naming plants in Latin. Every plant name in Latin is composed of two words like our first name and surname, the first name represents its genus (representing a particular family group) and second is the name of its species (which represents plants having similar properties, may or may not be from same geographical region). The classification of plants is called taxonomy, which categorizes them into division, class, order, family, genus and species. This process takes into account a number of factors, geographical, climatic conditions, type of plant its stem, number, shape, and position of leaves on the stem, shape and position of flowers, the number and shape of petals, whether the plant is hairy, prickly or smooth and so on.

If an essential oil is labeled and known, only by its common name, not only can incorrect use of a powerful, possibly hazardous oil abound but ignorance can result in a friendly oil being labeled as harmful. Latin names may sound intimidating but they are the best way to ensure what is in the bottle of essential oil.

PLANT FAMILIES :
Knowing a plant family is very helpful as plants of the same family have certain common therapeutic properties. As in case of Umbelliferae family having Thyme, Fennel, Carrot, Coriander etc, all of these plants have digestive and carminative properties. Here is a list of ten plant families covering almost sixty plants whose essential oils are used for aromatherapy.

Burseraceae (Resin Family)- Plants from this family exude resins; grown mostly in tropical desert, common examples are Frankincense, Myrrh, Elemi, Benzoin, Galbanum etc. These bring heat, contain energy to move fluids, heal wounds and build immune system besides being excellent meditational aid.

Compositae (Sun Flower Family)- Most of the plants from the Compositae family are known to be healers, anti inflammatory, sedating to nerves and emotions common examples are Chamomile, Immortelle (Helicrysm), Tagets , Davana etc.

Coniferae / Pinaceae (Pine Family)- Plants from this family are Pine, Juniper, Cypress, Cedar etc. giving oil from wood, needles or cones/berries etc. They are all strong antiseptics, astringent, diuretic, may also irritate skin, if used neat.

Graminnae (Grass Family)- Grasses give oils which are antiseptics, uplifting or grounding, bactericidal and immune builder; common examples are Lemongrass, Citronella, Palmarosa, Vertiver.

Labiatae (Mint Family)- All the oils from the plants of Mint family are therapeutic by nature, highly odorous they ease breathing, besides being carminative, immune builder and mood elevators. Common examples are Basil, Peppermint, Spearmint, Sage, Rosemary, Lavendin etc.

Lauracea (Laurel Family)- Common examples are Cassia, Bay, Rosewood, Camphor, Cinnamon etc. giving oils from wood bark or leaves, which are heating, stimulating and enhance memory.

Myrtaceae (Myrtle Family)- Commonly known plants are Eucalyptus, Tea Tree, Clove, Cajeput, Myrtle, Niaouli, Nutmeg etc, all known for their excellent therapeutic effect, they are good antiseptic, decongestant and immune builder.

Rutaceae (Citrus Family)- This family is known for its fruits and flowers, comprises of Lemon, Lime, Grapefruit, Orange, Bergamot, Mandarin, Tangerine etc. Oils from these plants are highly uplifting, enriching and invigorating.

Umbelliferae (Carrot Family)- Another therapeutically important plant family comprising of Carrots, Coriander, Fennel, Anise, Thyme, Cumin, Caraway, Parsley and Angelica; renowned for its digestive and carminative effect, they are good stimulants, digestive tonics, detoxifiers and decongestant.

Zingiberaceae (Ginger Family)- Turmeric, cardamom, Ginger are well known representative of this family, these are spice, root or fruit oils which increase circulation and heat, known as good antiseptics and digestive stimulants.

The following is a list of important essential oils commonly used in aromatherapy along with their detailed profiles followed by brief profiles of other essential oils, not so common in their use.

Note-The predicted benefits of Essential Oils mentioned in this chapter are not so much based on conventional scientific study as on observations of practitioners over many years of practice. Although some essential oils have undergone laboratory testing many more are yet to be examined scientifically.

Please note most of the plant oils are known for one or two specific properties which can be used at all the systems and organs of the body, if that can be remembered their use in practice becomes easy. To remember them easily, mark those properties and list them against each plants name, once you have gone through them. A word of advice to the beginners, please go through the cautions indicated for each oil, if any, then mark it on a label and stick to the essential oil bottle, so that every time you use the bottle of essential oil, you get reminded of the precaution you need to take while using the same oil.

Profiles

of

Important Essential Oils

Used in

Aromatherapy

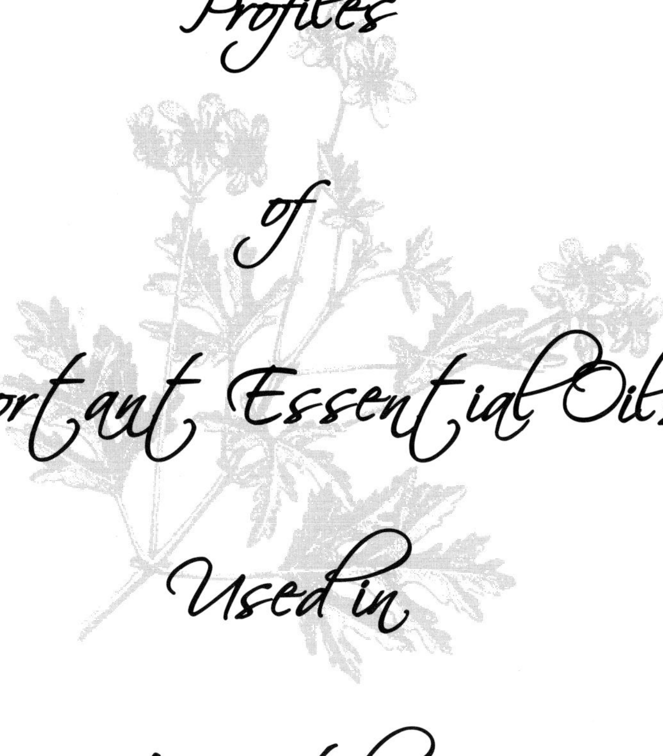

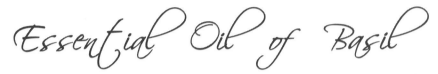

Essential Oil of Basil

(Ocimum basilicum / sanctum- Labiatae)

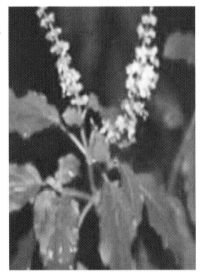

There are several variants of Basil, the one grown in India called Tulsi is highly revered in spiritual practice considered to be Sattvic (energy of purity) it is known as Holy Basil (Ocimum sanctum), widely used in Ayurvedic medicine and healing work. It is known to cleanse the aura, open heart Chakra, promotes detachment and brings clarity to mind. Other variants like European or sweet Basil (Ocimum basilicum), more used as culinary herb, contain a higher percentage of methyl chavicol.

Part of the plant used: Leaves, flowering tops

Method of extraction: Steam distillation

Volatility: Top Note

Principal Constituents: Camphor, cineol, phenol methyl ether, estragol (or methyl chavicol), eugenol, linalool and pinene.

Properties, effects and methods of use

Basil is a pale yellow liquid with, fresh, sweet-spicy scent, with balsamic undertone. It's odor effect is at first stimulating, giving way to a warm, comforting feeling. Basil is an effective diaphoretic (induces perspiration) also febrifuge(reduces fever), in most colds, flu and lungs problems. It is mostly used as a culinary herb, may be taken as a beverage with honey for promoting clarity of mind.

Emotional: Basil is a good fortifier of the nervous system, helps in mental tiredness, fatigue, anxiety and depression. It is particularly useful as a remedy for migraine.

Skin: Fresh leaf juice is used externally for fungal infections on the skin.

Digestive: Basil acts as a tonic and antispasmodic, considered to be good carminative, galactogenic and stomachic. It is also effective for travel sickness and nausea.

Circulatory: Basil stimulates circulation, clears skin congestion too.

Respiratory: Basil is effective remedy for asthma, bronchitis, nasal polyps and sinusitis.

Muscular: Basil oil is also useful for muscular aches and pains.

Gynecological: Basil is emmenagogic, regulates menstrual cycle, it can also be massaged, in a combination, on the solar plexus to control anxiety and menopausal symptoms.

Caution: Avoid during pregnancy; not to be used on sensitive skin; use in the lowest concentrations. It should only be used as a room scent due to its potentially irritant effect.

Essential Oil of Carrots

(Daucus Carota- umbelliferae)

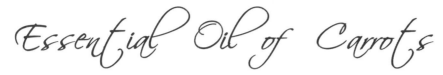

Carrots have become one of the world's most important root vegetables and are rich in nutritive and curative properties. In France, in the sixteenth century, carrots were prescribed as a remedy because of their carminative, stomachic and hepatic properties, they were grated and used on ulcers and have been thought of as blood cleanser, as a panacea for liver and skin problems.

Part of the plant used: Seeds

Method of extraction: Expression

Volatility: Middle note

Principal constituents: Acetic acid, alephatic aldehyde- arotal, Beta carotene, cineol, Formic acid, limonene, pinene, and terpineol.

Properties, effects and methods of use

Carrots are very useful in preparing for the Sun, particularly extra sensitive skins. They help prevent dryness, burns and the very early stages of cancer. For two months before going on a sunshine holiday, drink some carrot juice everyday for skin protection. You can also use the pulp from the juiced carrots as a mask once a week on any skin that needs moisturizing.

Skin-Carrots and carrot oil is good for skin; it is known for its blood cleansing properties, it clears up spots and blemishes. For aging skin, wrinkles and a bad color formulations used twice a year, for once a month each time will give elasticity, firmness and a good color. Macerated carrot oil can be used as base for facial formulations. While carrot seed oil is good for eczema and other skin infections.

Digestive-Carrots contain many important vitamins and minerals, vitamin A and Carotene, B-complex plus vitamins C,D,E and K, minerals, copper, iron, magnesium, manganese, phosphorous, potassium and sulphur. It also contains easily digestible sugar - levulose and dextrose. Carrots are goods for liver problems, diarrhea, constipation, anemia and rheumatism.

Circulatory- Carrot seed oil is useful for low blood pressure and hypotension.

Nervous System- It is a good neuro -tonic effective for nervous weakness and neurasthenia.

Gynaecological -Carrots are eaten during lactation to help to stimulate a good flow of milk.

Caution- *Carrot seed oil should be avoided on persons having high blood pressure.*

Essential Oil of Cedarwood

(Cedrus atlantica- Coniferae)

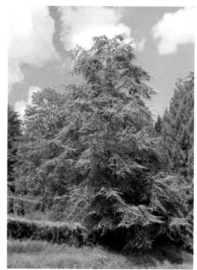

Cedrus or true cedar is the genus of four species of evergreen coniferous, hardy and long-lived trees. Cedrus atlantica, the Atlantic or Atlas cedar, is native to Atlas Mountains of Morocco, Cedrus Libani; the cedar of Lebanon is native to Syria and the Southeast Turkey; Cedrus libani var brevifollia comes from Cyprus; and Cedrus deodara, the deodar, comes from the Himalayas. Cedars are the trees most mentioned in the Bible, symbolizing everything that was fertile and abundant. The wood and its oil were used in embalming ancient Egyptians. For therapeutic use the only recognized oil of cedar is that from the Atlantic or Atlas Cedar or Atlas deodara.

Part of the plant used: Wood

Method of extraction: Steam Distillation

Volatility: Middle note

Principal constituents: Terpenic hydrocarbons, a little cedrol (which crystallizes when isolated) and sesquiterpenes (50%), especially cadinene and cedrene.

Properties, effects and methods of use

Cedarwood has effective therapeutic action on the scalp and in France it is included in commercial shampoos and hair lotions for alopecia. Over the last one hundred years, cedarwood's beneficial effects on the skin are noted and it's highly valued in dermatology. Woody aroma of the oil is considered a sexual stimulant, hence used in men's body preparations.

Skin- Cedarwood oil is quite effective for skin problems like eczema, dermatitis, seborrhea, rashes, skin eruptions and cellulite also.

Hair- Cedarwood oil is also well known for its therapeutic action for hair and scalp problems like alopecia, falling hair and dandruff. The oil has a tendency to darken hair color.

Caution- *Cedarwood has been prescribed internally in the past as a remedy for hemorrhoids, but stomach problems with intense burning sensations, thirst and nausea were recorded - so this oil is no more recommended to be taken internally.*

Essential Oil of German Chamomile

(Matricaria Chamomilla- Compositae / Asteraceae)

German Chamomile plants yield an oil with higher azulene content, which is used mainly to treat severe skin conditions.

Part of plant Used: Flowers

Methods of extraction: Steam distillation

Volatility: Middle note

Principal constituent: Sesquiterpenes chamazulene (less than 5 %), dihydro-chamazulkenes I and II, Bisabolenes, Sesquiterpenols, Sesquiterpininic oxides, Lactones and ethers.

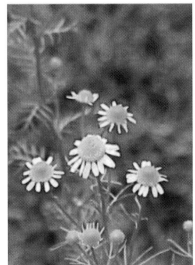

Properties, effects and methods of use

Essential oil of German Chamomile contains the powerful anti-inflammatory substance, azulene, which can relieve a wide variety of skin complaints.

Skin- Anti-inflammatory, soothing and antiseptic; good for sensitive and dry skins; helps to clear acne, eczema, psoriasis, diaper/nappy rash, burns, and minor wounds; reduces inflammations. Used in masks, compresses, application, or massage.

Digestive-Antispasmodic and anti-inflammatory; soothes diarrhea, dyspepsia, indigestion, flatulence, and colic; restores appetite. Used in compresses, baths, application, or massage.

Muscular-Calming and mild analgesic; soothes muscular aches and cramps due to physical exertion; relieves inflammation and pain in rheumatism and arthritis. Used in compresses, baths, application, or massage.

Gynaecological- Soothing and antispasmodic; helps painful, heavy or irregular menstruation; relieves pre-menstrual syndrome and menopausal symptoms. It is also useful for cystitis. Used in compresses, baths, or application.

Caution- *May cause hypersensitivity if undiluted. Avoid in the first trimester of pregnancy. It may cause skin irritation in some people.*

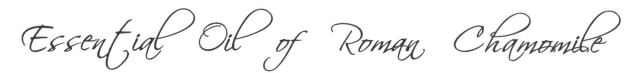

Essential Oil of Roman Chamomile

(Anthemis nobilis- Compositae / Asteraceae)

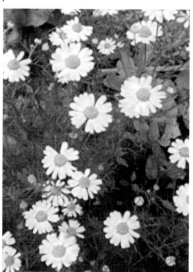

The small double flower heads of the cultivated variety of this species that are dried and then distilled to produce the high quality oil that is so valuable in aromatherapy practice.

Part of plant Used: Flowers

Methods of extraction: Steam distillation

Volatility: Middle note

Principal constituent: Esters (75-80%), monoterpinic alcohols (5-6%), ketone-pinocarvone.

Properties, effects and methods of use

Essential oil of Roman Chamomile oil, is highly valued in aromatherapy, has multiple healing properties and a low toxicity that make it particularly suitable for use on children. Roman chamomile has a light but sharp, apple-like aroma having a calming effect on central nervous system.

Emotional-Calming and relaxing; relieves anxiety, stress, depression, hysteria, irritability, and neuralgia; helpful in overcoming neurogenic shock, headaches and insomnia; soothing for children's tantrums. Used in inhalations, vaporizers, baths, application, or massage. Useful pre anaesthetic, prevents post operative shock.

Skin-Soothing and antiseptic, good for sensitive and dry skins; helps to clear acne, eczema, diaper/nappy rash, burns, allergies, and minor wounds; reduces inflammations. Used in masks, compresses, application, or massage.

Digestive-Antispasmodic; anti parasitic, soothes diarrhea, dyspepsia, nausea, indigestion, flatulence, and colic; restores appetite. Used in compresses, baths, application, or massage.

Muscular-Calming and mild analgesic; soothes muscular aches and cramps due to physical exertion; relieves inflammation and pain in rheumatism and arthritis. Used in compresses, baths, application, or massage.

Gynaecological- Soothing and antispasmodic; helps painful, heavy or irregular menstruation; relieves pre-menstrual syndrome and menopausal symptoms Used in compresses, baths, or application.

Essential Oil of Clary Sage

(Saivia sclarea- Labiatae)

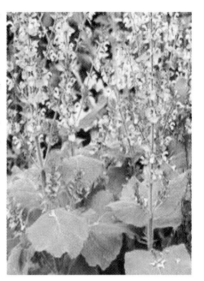

This beautiful plant is to be found growing high up in the Alps, wherever the soil is loose and dry. Small blue or white flowers grow out of large, pinky mauve bracts. Branches of these bracts radiate out in pairs from a spectacular central stem that reaches a height of 60 inches (1.5m). The powerful aroma of Clary Sage, somewhat resembles that of Muscatel wine; in the past, German winemakers used the herb to improve cheap wines. Clary Sage bears no resemblance to Common, or Garden Sage, Salvia officianalis, which yields an entirely different essential oil.

Part of plant used: Flowering tops

Method of extraction: Steam distillation

Volatility: Top note

Principal constituents: Linalol, linalyl acetate, sclareol and terpenic esters.

Properties, effects, and methods of use

Clary Sage is a neurotonic, powerful relaxant, and a sedative essential oil. It has a pervading, sweet, sensuous aroma that can be quite heady. The oil is known as 'women's best friend', as it is good for all hormonal imbalances, PMS and menopausal symptoms.

Emotional-Uplifting and relaxing; helpful in relieving depression, anxiety, tension, mental fatigue, and general debility; it is an effective sedative- promotes profound, dreams filled sleep; good for calming cross or irritable children. Used in inhalations, vaporizers, bath, application, or massage.

Respiratory-Calming and anti-inflammatory; relieves sore throats and hoarseness. Used in inhalations, vaporizes, or application.

Circulatory-Effective remedy for hypertension the oil is Calming; reduces high blood pressure. Used in inhalations, vaporization, compresses, baths, or massage.

Gynecological-Antispasmodic, anti-inflammatory, and a gentle menstrual stimulant; relieves amenorrhea, dysmenorrhea, premenstrual syndrome and menstrual pain; helps to establish menstrual regularity; soothes swollen breasts; relieve / prevent hot flushes. Used in compresses, baths, or massage.

Caution: *Since inhalation of the oil may cause sleepiness, keep to recommended dosages and use for short periods only, preferably at the end of the day when no further physical or mental exertion is required. Do not combine with alcohol, or inhale before driving. Avoid use during first five months of pregnancy.*

Essential Oil of Cypress

(Cupressus sempervirens- Cupresaceae/ Coniferae)

The elegant, graceful form of this tree is a feature of the landscape of southern France where, traditionally, it is planted in graveyards. Today, C. semepervirens is commercially cultivated for its oil in, both, Germany and France. In the past, the Egyptians used Cypress wood to make the coffins in which they placed their mummies, while the ancient Chinese believed in the healing properties of the tree, chewing on the fruit to prevent bleeding gums and loss of teeth.

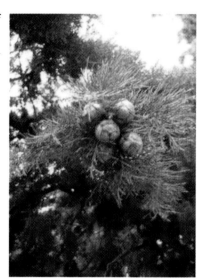

Part of plant used: Twigs, needles, and cones

Method of extraction: Steam distillation

Volatility: Middle note

Principal constituents: Monoterpenes-Pinene & carene, sesquiterpenes and sesquiterpinol-cedrol and diterpinic acids.

Properties, effects, and methods of use

Essential oil of Cypress is primarily beneficial to the circulatory and vascular systems. It is also known for it's astringent and styptic properties (the later causes constriction of blood vessels and helps to prevent blood loss).

Emotional-Sedative and soothing: helps to clear the mind of grief and prepare it for sleep; useful against insomnia. It can be used in vaporizers, baths, application, or massage.

Respiratory-Antispasmodic and antiseptic; relieves spasmodic and whooping coughs, useful for asthma and laryngitis. Used in gargles, inhalations, vaporizers, baths or application.

Skin- Useful for oily skin, as an astringent, effective for open pores, it can be used in flower waters, cleansers or facial massage.

Circulatory-Astringent and styptic; relieves fluid retention and cellulite; invaluable in the treatment of bleeding gums, edema of lower limbs, varicose veins, hemorrhoids, circulatory cramps/chilblains and broken capillaries. Can be used in bath or skin application.

Digestive- Helps in diarrhea, nausea and dyspepsia.

Muscular-Tonic; helpful for cramps; reduces swelling in rheumatism. Used in baths, compresses, application, or massage.

Gynecological-Antispasmodic and styptic; can help to staunch a hemorrhage or excessive blood loss; relieves painful menstruation and menopausal spotting; useful after childbirth as a means of controlling the amount of blood lost and for calming vulval tissues. Used in compresses, baths, application, or massage.

Caution: *Avoid using if you suffer from high blood pressure.*

Essential Oil of Eucalyptus

(Eucalyptus globules- Myrtaceae)

Of the various species of Eucalyptus native to Australia and Tasmania, only a small number are grown for their essential oil. During the heat of summer, Eucalyptus trees appear surrounded by a blue haze, as essential oil evaporates from their leaves, releasing antiseptic properties that may help to protect against blight and pests. The term the "blue forests of Australia" originates in this phenomenon. Today, Eucalyptus trees are grown successfully in many sub-tropical countries include Spain, Portugal, India, Zimbabwe and China.

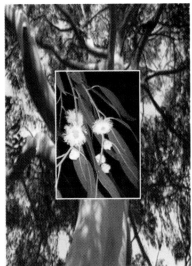

Part of plant used: Leaves

Method of extraction: Steam distillation

Volatility: Top note

Principal constituents: An oxide - Cineol or Eucalyptol (60-80%), along with various aldehydes, ketones, sesquiterpinic alcohols and terpenes.

Properties, effects and methods of use

Essential oil of Eucalyptus is strong natural antiseptic that may be effective against a wide range of bacterial and viral infections. It has an overall cooling effect on the body and is useful in reducing fevers. The oil is clear with a strong camphoraceous smell that makes it a good anti catarrhal and decongestant besides a good insect repellant.

Emotional- Uplifting and invigorating; clears and stimulates the mind and helps to prevent drowsiness. Used in inhalations, vaporizers, baths application, or massage.

Respiratory- Antiseptic and decongestant; helps to fight and prevent colds, flu, throat infections, sinusitis, and headaches caused by congestion; eases tight, dry coughs; relieves the breathlessness of asthma and bronchitis by loosening mucus. Used in gargles, inhalations, vaporizers, baths, application, or massage.

Skin- Cooling and antiseptic; effective in the treatment of bacterial / fungal dermatitis, boils, pimples, head lice, and herpes simplex. Used in compresses or application.

Circulatory-Cleansing and detoxifying, it stimulates and strengthens the kidneys. Used in baths, massage or application.

Muscular- Anti-inflammatory, reduces swelling and helps to relieve muscular aches and pains, rheumatism, and arthritis. Can be used in compresses, bath, application, or massage.

Urinary-Eucalyptus oil also help to alleviate cystitis, when used in sitz bath.

Caution-*Once absorbed into the bloodstream, Eucalyptus oil can irritate the kidneys or skin if used in too high concentrations-avoid using on small children.*

Essential Oil of Frankincense

(Boswellia carteri- Burseraceae)

One of the three gifts from Magi to child Jesus, Frankincense has been used since olden times in churches also for other religious/ spiritual rituals, cleansing. Also known as Olibanum this aromatic gum resin obtained, in Africa, Middle East, and various Indian regions, from trees of the genus Boswellia, mainly B. Carteri.

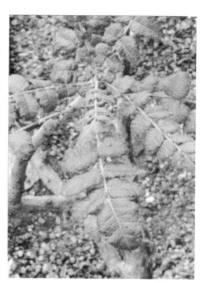

Part of plant used: Gum exudes

Extraction: Steam distillation or solvent extraction

Volatility: Middle note

Principal constituents: Monoterpene alpha & beta pinene, limonene, sesquiterpine, terpinic alcohols, Ketonic alcohol (olibbanol).

Properties effects and methods of use

A colorless to pale yellow liquid with a warm, balsamic fragrance, subtly lemony, and sometimes with a note of camphor. The odor improves greatly as the oil ages. The odor effect is warming and balancing to the emotions. The oil is considered to be immunostimulant.

Emotional/ Mental- Frankincense is used in religious rituals and as a major ingredient in church rituals, it is a meditational aid, helps to maintain a clear mind and preserves spiritual energy. It relieves nervous depression, stress and anxiety.

SKIN: Due to its rejuvenating properties Frankincense is useful in skin care particularly mature skin, scars, wounds.

Respiratory: Useful for respiratory ailments, asthma, bronchitis, colds and flu.

Gynecological: Frankincense is also a mild hormone regulator, helps in dysmenorrhea, menorrhagnia besides being useful in treatment of leucorrhoea and cystitis.

Digestive : It has been found to be useful in dyspepsia and flatulence.

Caution: *May cause skin irritation in some people.*

Essential Oil of Geranium

(Pelargonium graveolens- Geraniaceae)

A native of Africa, the Geranium plant was brought to Europe in the late 17th century. There are now more than 700 species, of which P. graveolens and P. odoratissimum are the ones commonly used in aromatherapy. The centre for commercial cultivation of Geranium is the island of Reunion in the Indian Ocean, although France, Spain, Italy, Morocco, Egypt and China are also Producers, the best quality comes from Ooty in South India.

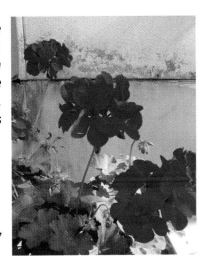

Part of plant used: Leaves

Method of extraction: Steam distillation

Volatility: Middle note

Principal constituents: Mono & Sesqui terpinols, Geraniol, citronellol, linalool and terpinic esters with traces of oxides, ketones and terpenes.

Properties, effect, and methods of use

Essential oil of Geranium is a good all-rounder. It is anti infectious, antibacterial, antifungal, antispasmodic and lymphatic tonic. It is effective in cleansing the body and uplifting the mind. The oil has a rich, sweet aroma and is usually greenish-yellow in color.

Emotional-Highly versatile uplifting as well as relaxing depending on the combination of other oils it is used with, useful against stress; alleviates depression and anxiety. Used in inhalations, vaporizers, baths, application, or massage.

Respiratory-Cleansing and calming; helps to fight colds and flu; relieves throat and mouth infections Used in mouthwashes or gargles.

Skin-Astringent and balancing; cleanses and tones the skin and normalizes secretion of sebum; reduces inflammation; relieves acne, fungal dermatitis, dry eczema, head lice, dandruff, herpes simplex, stretch marks and minor wounds, soothes measles rashes in children. Used in baths or application.

Digestive -Tonic and cleansing; effective against mouth ulcers, diarrhea, and gastroenteritis. Used in compresses, baths, application, or massage.

Circulatory-Astringent, stimulant and antiseptic; assists elimination of' waste products, can help to relieve fluid retention and cellulite. Used in baths, application, or massage.

Gynaecological- Stimulant and regulator of hormone production; it is helpful for pre- menstrual syndrome, menopausal symptoms, vaginal infections, and sterility. Used in inhalations, compresses, baths, application, or massage.

Essential Oil of Juniperberry

Juniper (Juniperis communis- Coniferae)

Two types of essential oil are distilled from this evergreen shrub. Juniper Berry oil is the better quality of the two and the one recommended for aromatherapy use. It is distilled from little ripe berries that have been picked straight from the bush and dried, also used during distillation of gin, occasionally a poorer quality Juniper oil is produced by adding berries that have been partially distilled in the making of gin or by extracting oil from the berries, leaves, and branches. Both types are sold under the name of Juniper Berry oil.

Part of plant used: Ripe berries

Method of extraction: Steam distillation

Volatility: Middle note

Principal constituents: Alpha & Beta Pinene, Mono & Sesqui terpineol and terpinic esters.

Properties, effects and methods of use

Essential oil of Juniper Berry is noted primarily for its antiseptic and diuretic properties. The oil is colorless to pale yellow, when freshly distilled, but it grows darker and thicker with age. The fresh aroma is similar to that of Cypress (both plants are from the same family), but sharper and more peppery.

Emotional- Calming and tonic, hypotensive, helpful in overcoming anxiety and mental fatigue. Used in masks, compresses or application.

Skin- Astringent and cleansing, beneficial for acne, oily skin, greasy hair, dandruff,

and weeping eczema. Used in masks, compresses, or application.

Digestive- Antiseptic and gas/wind relieving; relieves indigestion, flatulence, diarrhea and colic. Used in baths, compresses, application, or massage.

Circulatory- Stimulant and excellent diuretic; helps to lower blood pressure; cleanses the body, relieving fluid retention, cellulite, varicose veins, and haemorrhoids; strengthens the kidneys. Used in baths, application or massage.

Muscular- Tonic and stimulant, useful for muscular aches/ pains and rheumatism. Used in compresses, baths, application or massage.

Gynecological- As a diuretic it is also helpful for irregular or painful menstruation; invaluable when breasts are swollen during menstruation. Used in compresses, bath, or application. Juniper Berry oil may also alleviate cystitis, when used in baths or application.

Caution: *Avoid use during first five months of pregnancy, and in cases of severe kidney disease, where once absorbed into the bloodstream, the oil can over stimulate the kidneys.*

Essential Oil of Lavender

(Lavandula officianalis /L. angustifolia or L. Vera- Labiatae)

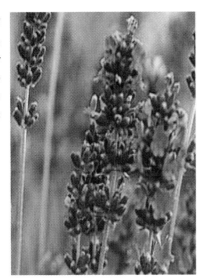

Much of our pure Lavender oil now comes from Yugoslavia and Bulgaria; France still produces the finest quality, but production there tumbled with the advent of the hybrid Lavendin which grows at low altitudes. True lavender thrives at around 3,000 ft (1,000 mtrs). It is the showy purple of Lavendin that transforms the landscape of southern France in summer however the subtle blue of true lavender is far less striking.

Part of plant used: Flowering tops

Method of extraction: Steam distillation

Volatility: Middle note

Principal constituents: Linalyl and Geranyl esters, geraniol, linalool.

Properties, Effects and Method of use

Lavender essential oil has a balancing and normalizing effect, bringing health and harmony to the body and mind. It is non-toxic, and has a full, flowery aroma.

Emotional-Uplifting and soothing; alleviates stress, anxiety, depression, and general debility; helpful for insomnia, headaches and migraine. Used in inhalations, vaporizers, compresses, baths application, or massage.

Respiratory- Antiseptic and anti-inflammatory; relieves colds, flu, sinusitis and throat infections. Used in inhalations, vaporizers, baths or application.

Skin-Balancing, antiseptic, anti-inflammatory, and regenerative; soothes acne, eczema, dandruff, hair loss, head lice, diaper/nappy rash, sunburn, insect bites, and boils; relieves athlete's foot and herpes simplex; effective for burns and stretch marks since it promotes cell growth and helps to minimize scarring. Used in masks, compresses, baths or application.

Digestive- Cleansing and calming; helps bad breath, mouth ulcers, indigestion, flatulence, nausea, and gastroenteritis. Used in compresses, application, or massage.

Circulatory-Sedative and decongestant; lowers blood pressure; reduces palpitations, alleviates fluid retention by assisting elimination of waste products through the lymphatic system. Used in baths, application, or massage.

Muscular- Analgesic and anti-inflammatory; helpful for muscular sprains, aches, pains and rheumatism. Used in compresses, baths, application, or massage.

Gynecological-Calming and balancing; helps to establish menstrual regularity, good for pre-menstrual and menopausal symptoms alleviates thrush. Used in compresses, inhalations, vaporizers, baths, or application.

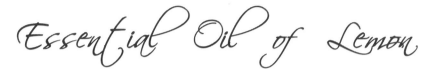
Essential Oil of Lemon

(Citrus limonum - Rutaceae)

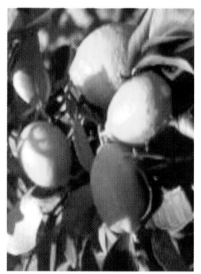

It is a relatively small member of the Citrus family. It originated in South East Asia, in India, China, Japan but is now grown extensively in hot countries around the Mediterranean, in Spain, Southern Italy, Sicily and the South of France. Although small, an individual tree can produce up to 1,500 lemons per year. Lemon essential oil is called "polyvalent" (cure-all) by French phyto therapists.

Part of the plant used: Oily rind of the fruit

Method of extraction: Cold expression

Volatility: Top note

Principal constituents: Limonene (upto 90%) and Citral (3 to 5%)

Properties, effects and Methods of use

The therapeutic values of lemon took time to get recognized. Nicholas Lewery, in his book on simple drugs in 1968, mentioned them. They were classified as digestive, as a blood cleanser and as helping sweeten the breath after a heavy meal. They reached the height of their therapeutic fame when they were issued to counteract the effects of scurvy on the British Navy, (resulting in the erroneous nickname of limey).

Emotional-Stimulating, uplifting and invigorating; it acts to sharpen mind and restore or increase vitality. Used in inhalations, baths (am) or application.

Digestive-It is a tonic, stimulant, stomachic, carminative helps relieve dyspepsia and gastritis.

Respiratory-Lemon is a well known and popular remedy for colds, bronchitis and laryngitis.

Skin-Cooling and cleansing acts as simple pore-refining toner used on greasy skin and blockheads. Soothes itchy skin it helps in psoriasis. Also makes for a good hair rinser for oily scalp, clears dandruff.

Circulatory-Lemon improves circulation, is useful for all vein problems, varicose or broken capillaries.

Gynecological-Lemon also helps the symptoms of premenstrual tensions and insomnia. This is also good for stomach skin during pregnancy, for the breasts and the nipples, improving circulation all around.

Caution- *Lemon oil should be used fresh, as it gets oxidized soon if left open or in the light. Oxidized oil can cause terrible allergic reaction (old oxidized oil will look cloudy - so discard if cloudy). Since Lemon is photosensitive it should not be used prior to sunbathing or before going out in the sun.*

Essential Oil of Marjoram (Sweet)

(Origanum marjorana- Labiatae)

Marjoram is thought to have originated in Asia, but it is being grown in all over Europe. The plant was sacred to Shiva and Vishnu (Indian deities) and to Osiris in Egypt. To Greeks it was Amarakos, a symbol of love and honor. Aphrodite used to cure her son Aeneas wounds, apparently it was scentless till she touched it.

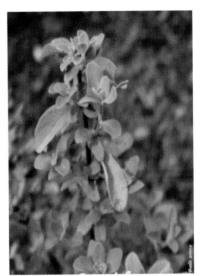

Part of the plant used: Flowers

Method of extraction: Steam distillation

Volatility: Middle note

Principal constituents: Phenols 80% (carvacrol and thymol) with borneol, camphor, cineol, cymene, pinene, sabinene and terpineol.

Properties, effects and Methods of use

A pale yellow liquid with a warm spicy - camphoraceous aroma. Its odor effect is warming and calming; it is reputed to quell sexual desire. Marjoram has been in use as an oil, as well as, a herb, it's a stomachic, expectorant and sedative particularly useful when you are tired or suffering from insomnia.

Emotional : Marjoram calms and sedates the nerves, it is good for treating insomnia, migraines, nervous tension and tension headaches.

Skin : Useful in ointments for bruises, also in hair formulations to maintain natural colour and lustre of hair and brows.

Digestive : Marjoram is effective in stomach disorders, flatulence and stomach pain.

Respiratory: Eases asthma, bronchitis, colds, coughs and snoring.

Muscular : Relieves chill pains, muscular stiffness and spasmic pains.

Gynecological : Useful in relieving conditions of painful menstruation, absence of menstruation outside pregnancy and PMS. Quells sexual desire.

Caution: *Not to be used during pregnancy. It may cause skin irritation in sensitive people.*

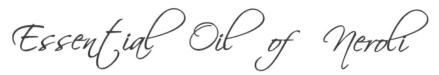

Essential Oil of Neroli

(Citrus aurantium bigaradia var amara- Rutaceae)

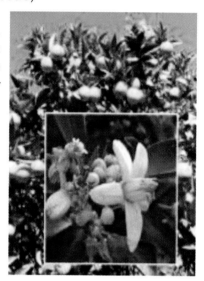

Neroli essential oil is extracted by distillation of Orange (Bitter) flowers, though solvent extracted absolutes are also available. The main commercial producers are Italy, France, Egypt and Sicily, however the best oil comes from Tunisia and Sicily, orange flower water is the by product of distillation process.

Part of the plant used: Flowers

Method of extraction: Steam distillation

Volatility: Middle note

Principal constituents: Acetic esters, dipentene, terpineol, farnesol, geraniol, indol, jasmone, l-camphene, alpha & beta pinene, nerol, nerolidol

Properties, effects and Methods of use

The essential oil is pale yellow liquid with a sweet, floral fragrance with bitter and sour undertone. The absolute is dark amber viscous liquid with a fresh warm, sweet-floral fragrance, very similar to the scent of fresh orange blossom. The aroma effect of both neroli and orange flower absolute is uplifting, calming and antidepressant; a reputed aphrodisiac.

Emotional: Neroli is a good relaxing as well as uplifting oil. It gives confidence and strength to mind, has relaxing properties and has slightly hypnotic effect which helps with sleeplessness.

Skin: Neroli is good for mature skin also helpful in inflammation, dermatitis and broken capillaries.

Respiratory: Neroli oil helps in bronchitis, respiratory disorders and pulmonary TB.

Digestive: Neroli helps in digestive problems like flatulence, entrocolitis and regulates liver and pancreatic malfunctions.

Gynecological : Neroli has a special affinity to female immune system , it helps women in any stage of transition, reduces cramps and assists in menopause.

Caution: *Because of its high price petit grain is often added to Neroli, which reduces the therapeutic effect of the oil.*

Essential Oil of Palmarosa

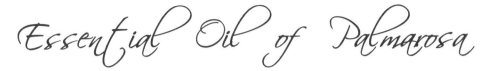

(Cymbopogon martini-Gramineae)

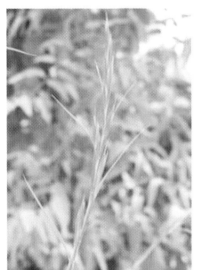

It belongs to a family of tropical grasses rich in aromatic, volatile oils, formerly known mostly under the generic name of Andropogon, but now included in the genus cymbopogon. Originally from Central and Northern India, and now cultivated in Africa and Madagascar as well, the grass is slender, bearing panicles of blue-white color that mature to dark red.

Part of the plant used: Leaves & Flowers

Method of extraction: Steam Distillation

Volatility: Top note

Principal constituent: Monoterpinic alcohols mainly Gernaniol (between 75 and 90%) and esters.

Properties, effects and methods of use

The plant has long been used in India, also called poor man's Geranium, it is taken internally as a remedy against infection and fever. A high proportion of geraniol in the oil makes it a natural antiseptic and bactericidal. Palmarosa can relieve discomforts of flu and high temperature, also helps in MS (Multiple Sclerosis).

Emotional- Palmarosa has comparatively mild odor having relaxing effect on the mind; like Geranium it is quite versatile and becomes relaxing in combination with relaxing oils and uplifting in combination with uplifting oils.

Skin- Wonderful remedy for skin conditions like acne because of its natural antiseptic constituents, also works wonderfully for boils (apply directly), for old acne scars, for wrinkles specially those occurring after long exposure to the sun. It is also useful for hair loss and dandruff control.

Circulatory - Wonderful remedy for broken veins.

Methods of use - Bath (a.m.) massage, compresses & application.

Essential Oil of Patchauli

(Pogostomon cablin - Labiatae)

The essential oil is obtained from the leaves and young shoots of herbaceous shrub native to Malaysia, where it is called cablin. It is now cultivated in many places, including India (where it is known as patcha or patchapat), Indonesia, Seychelles, and China. It grows to about three feet in height, and when rubbed the fresh leaves yield the characteristic earthy and woody smell of patchauli. The antiseptic properties of Patchauli were studied in 1922 by Gati and Cayola, by Sarbach in 1962 and by many other well known scientists.

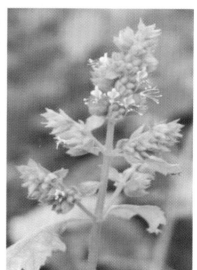

Part of the plant used: Leaves and shoots

Method of extraction: Steam Distillation

Volatility: Middle note

Principal constituents: Patchoulol and sesquiterpettes

Properties, effects and methods of use

Patchauli has always played a large part in the traditional Malay, Chinese and Japanese medicine, being attributed as a stimulant, bactericidal, effective against fever, epidemics and many other illnesses, it also helps in skin rejuvenation and used as remedy for snake venom and insect bite. Patchauli has a great part to play in perfumery as it acts as a natural fixative, reinforcing the woody note of perfume giving it even greater intensity.

Emotional- Relieves anxieties, tension, restore emotional balance; it is helpful in freeing the mind from past. Being a base note oil it is used as a natural fixative since its earthy smell lasts longer and becomes quite sensual in combination with the body chemistry, it has also been mentioned in Kama Sutras. It can be used in inhalations, vaporizers, baths and applications or massage.

Skin- Patchauli is a good tissue regenerator, recommended for many skin conditions; allergies, herpes, impetigo, bed sores, burns, cracked skin, haemorrhoids and eczema.

Circulatory- Patchauli is helpful in treatment of hemorrhoids and varicose veins.

Digestive- Patchauli is a good digestive, stomachic helps in irritable bowel and entrocolitis.

Caution- Patchauli may sometimes be adulterated with cubeb and cendar oils. Unless you are sure of the purity of the oils do not use them therapeutically.

Essential Oil of Peppermint

(Mentha piperita- Lamiaceae / Labiatae)

Commercially cultivated on a wide scale in Europe, USA, and Japan, Peppermint oil is used extensively in the toiletry, food, and pharmaceutical industries. A variety of products ranging from toothpastes, mouthwashes, and digestive tablets to candy sweets, ice cream and liquors are flavored with Peppermint. Comparatively aromatherapy makes use of only a minute proportion (possibly less than 1%) of the annual worldwide output of Peppermint essential oil.

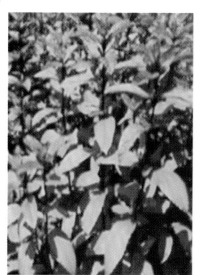

Part of plant used: Leaves

Method of extraction: Steam distillation

Volatility: Top note

Principal constituents: Monoterpinic alcohols mainly Menthol (38-48%), Ketones mainly menthone(20-30%), some monoterpenes and oxides.

Properties, effects, and methods of use

Essential oil of Peppermint promotes overall physical and emotional well being, although its healing properties are primarily associated with the digestive system. It is a good antiseptic, antibacterial and antiviral. It has a light, clean, refreshing aroma, and is a good insect repellant.

Emotional- Stimulating and strengthening; uplifts the system and is especially useful in the treatment of shock; helpful for neuralgia and relief of general debility, headaches and migraines. Used in inhalations, baths or application.

Respiratory- Antiseptic and antispasmodic; effective in reducing mucus and relieving coughs, sinusitis, throat infections, colds, flu, asthma and bronchitis. Used in inhalations, baths, or application.

Skin- Cooling and cleansing; sooths itchy skin; relieves inflammation.

Digestive- Soothing and antispasmodic; relieves acidity, heartburn, diarrhea, indigestion, and flatulence; also highly effective for travel sickness and nausea; helps to combat bad breath. Used in gargles or application.

Circulatory- Having a Cooling effect the oil is also helpful for varicose veins and hemorrhoids. Used in compresses or application.

Gynecological- Cooling and decongestant; encourages menstrual regularity; relieves hot flushes. Used in baths, application, or massage.

Caution: *Too concentrated a dose of Peppermint oil can cause itchiness- keep to recommended dilutions. Keep your eyes closed when inhaling. Avoid use if you suffer from epilepsy or other neural*

Essential Oil of Rose

(Rose damascana or centifolia-Rosaceae)

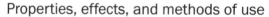

Rose is a native of orient, it is now being cultivated almost all over the world. It is highly regarded though it is one of the most difficult oil to extract. It is solvent extracted, as well as, steam distilled. In traditional extraction process almost two tonnes of Rose petals are required to get a kilo of Rose oil, there is hardly any oil in the first distil, so the distilled water along with oil has to be recycled with fresh petals to increase oil concentration, the ultimate result is a distillers dream- ROOH(Life Force) GULAB, considered as the best quality oil. However Bulgarian Rose oil and absolutes are also quite popular in Europe and American continent. Rose water the by product, of steam distillation, has been used since ages in skin and beauty care as well as flavoring.

Part of the plant used: Flower Petals

Method of extraction: Steam distillation

Volatility: Middle note

Principal constituents: Eugenol, farnesol and other acids, geraniol (or citronellol), linalool, nerol, nonylic aldehydes, rhodinol and stearoptene.

Properties, effects, and methods of use

Rose is a highly valued essential oil, it alleviates depression, gives a sense of security and spiritual attunement. It heals and keeps your heart open and connected to all things. It is said a drop of rose oil applied to heart chakra helps in breast cancer. It reduces anger and strengthens liver function, it is natures gift to women and alleviates menopausal symptoms. Rose has also been prescribed for frigidity therefore ascribing aphrodisiac properties to it.

Emotional : Rose essential oil is very good for people with nervous disposition. Its odour effect is calming, uplifting and antidepressant. It is a reputed aphrodisiac.

SKIN : Rose essential oil and Rose water had been traditionally used for skin and beauty care, particularly for mature skin. Rose water or infusions are also useful for eye wash, eyelid complaints as well as skin ulcers.

Respiratory : Rose has also been found valuable for respiratory problems like coughs, hay fever, sinus congestion and bronchitis.

Digestive : Rose is a mild laxative and helps in symptoms of anorexia and loss of appetite.

Gynecological: Rose is considered to be an aphrodisiac, helps in frigidity, premenstrual tension and menopausal symptoms.

Caution: In spite of its gentle nature Rose oil may sometimes irritate the skin due to small percentage of

Essential Oil of Rosemary

(Rosmarinus officinalis- Labiatae/ Lamiaceae)

The common name for this plant, Rosemary, comes from the Latin Rosmarinus which means "dew of the sea". Bushes of this aromatic herb are to be found growing wild in Mediterranean regions, often quite close to the sea shore. Its history dates back to its use by the ancient Egyptians, and its revered status symbol of love and death, in the religious ceremonies and funeral rites of the ancient Greeks and Romans. Therapeutically, it has been in use for hundreds of years, valued for its antiseptic and invigorating properties.

Part of the plant used: Flowering tops

Method of extraction: Steam distillation

Volatility: Top note

Principal constituents: Cineol, borneol, pinene

Properties, effects, and methods of use

Essential oil of Rosemary is noted for its strongly antiseptic and stimulating properties. It is also a gentle analgesic and regulator that helps to balance body and mind. It has a slightly camphoraceous, warm, pungent aroma.

Emotional- Stimulating and astringent; stimulates the memory, clears the mind, and helps to relieve headaches, migraines, and general fatigue. Used in inhalations, vaporizers, baths, application, or massage.

Respiratory- Antiseptic and antispasmodic; relieves coughs, colds and flu. Used in inhalations, compresses, or massage.

Skin- Cleansing and stimulating; helps to prevent dandruff and hair loss. Used in rinses, application, or massage.

Digestive- Antiseptic and gas/wind relieving; helps indigestion, flatulence, constipation, colitis, gastroenteritis, and stomach pains; also stimulates the liver. Used in compresses, application, or massage.

Circulatory-Tonic and astringent; helps in low blood pressure, improve circulation, and reduce lymphatic congestion; relieves fluid retention, cellulite, and varicose veins. Used in baths, application or massage.

Muscular- Gentle analgesic without sedative effects; relieves general aches and pains, sprains, and arthritis. Used in compresses, application, or massage.

Gynecological- Stimulating and normalizing; helps to regulate the menstrual cycle. Used in baths, application, or massage.

Essential Oil of Sandalwood

(Santalum album- Santalaceae)

The centre of commercial cultivation of Sandalwood is Karnataka. From here comes the finest quality essential oil, distilled from the wood of fully mature trees. Sandalwood oil has long been in use in Ayurvedic medicine for its healing properties and reputed to improve the memory. It is also one of the oils mentioned in the Bible. King Solomon was told by God to use Sandalwood for the making of the furniture in his great temple. This he apparently did, and the temple was filled with the beautiful smell of the oil.

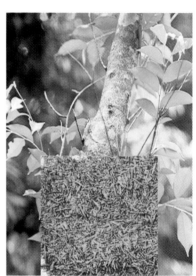

Part of plant used: Wood

Method of extraction: Steam distillation

Volatility: Base note

Principal constituents: Santalol (over 90%)

Properties, effects, and methods of use

Sandalwood oil is profoundly relaxing, calming, soothing and a good meditation aid. An excellent antiseptic for both pulmonary and urinary systems, with rich woody smell, making the oil, quite pleasant for therapeutic use.

Emotional- Calming, Sedative and relaxing; beneficial for relieving anxiety and depression; helpful in freeing the mind from the past; invaluable as a remedy for insomnia. Used in inhalations, vaporizers, baths, application, or massage.

Respiratory- Soothing and antiseptic; relieves irritation and soreness in chesty coughs, sore throats, and laryngitis; soothes inflammation in bronchitis and asthma. Used in gargles, inhalations, vaporizers, application, or massage.

Skin- Balancing and anti-inflammatory; softens dry, mature, or wrinkled skin; helps dry dandruff and eczema; reduces inflammation and irritation from sunburn, nettle rash, hives, diaper/nappy rash, and allergic conditions. Used in compresses, application, or massage.

Digestive- Calming and antispasmodic; subdues vomiting, colic and hiccups; helpful for diarrhea; soothes heartburn and nausea, especially morning sickness. Used in compresses, application or massage.

Circulatory- Soothing, relieves itchiness in hemorrhoids and varicose veins. Used in compresses or application.

Urinary- Sandalwood oil, would soothe cystitis and other urinary infections, when used in sitz baths

Gynecological- Hormone regulator and balancer, the oil is good for pre-menstrual and menopausal symptoms. Used in baths or application.

Essential Oil of Tea Tree

(Melaleuca alternifolia-Myrtaceae)

When Captian Cook and his sailors first visited the Australian continent, they were said to have used the leaves of this tree to make a refreshing hot drink. Whether or not they liked the brew is uncertain but the tree has kept the name they gave it. Over the centuries, the indigenous Aborigines have used Tea Tree poultices to cleanse and heal wounds and ulcers. Today it is grown commercially for its oil along the central and northern coasts of New South Wales.

Part of plant used: Leaves

Method of extraction: Steam distillation

Volatility: Top note

Principal constituents: Terpenes, terpinolene, terpinen-4-ol, terpineol

Properties, effects, and methods of use

Tea Tree essential oil is an exceptionally powerful antiseptic, being 12 times as strong as carbolic acid, or phenol, the widely used chemical disinfectant. It has the advantage of being both hypo-allergenic and non-toxic, and it may also be effective against a range of bacterial, viral, and fungal conditions. The oil can be pale green to almost water clear, and its aroma is an effective insect repellant.

Respiratory- Bactericidal and anti-viral; helps to fight colds and flu; alleviates sore throats, tonsillitis, and gum disease; eases bronchitis, chesty coughs, and congestion. Used in gargles, mouthwashes, compresses, inhalations, vaporizers, or application.

Skin- Cleansing, cooling and anti-fungal; relieves boils and rashes; soothes sunburn; encourages open skin to heal while protecting it from infection; relieves athlete's foot and nail bed infections. Used in masks, compresses, foot or hand baths, or application.

Digestive- Bactericidal, anti-viral, and anti-fungal; eases mouth ulcers; calms diarrhea and relieves gastroenteritis. Used in mouthwashes, compresses, application, or massage.

Gynaecological- Very effective for genital infections, specially leucorrhea, candida and thrush. Used in sitz baths, douches, baths, or application.

Caution: In spite of the fact that this oil can be used neat, it may sometimes cause sensitization of the skin.

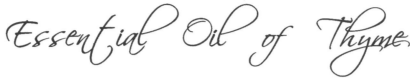

Essential Oil of Thyme

(Thymus Spp, T. citriodorits, T. vulgaris- Labiatae / Lamiaceae)

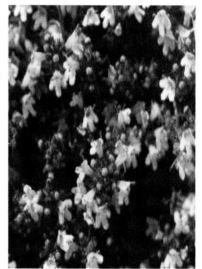

The name thyme actually comes from the Greek word thymos meaning smell, because of the fragarnce of the plant. Thyme belongs to a genus of over three hundred species of hardy, perennial herbaceous plants and shrubs that are native to Europe, particularly around Mediteranean. It is one of Hippocrates four hundred simple remedies.

Part of plant used: Leaves and flowering tops

Method of extraction: Steam distillation

Volatility: Top note

Principal constituents: 25 -40% thymol and carvacrol with borneol, cineol, linalool, menthone, B-cymene, pinene and triterpenic acid

Properties, effects and method of use

Thyme had been used differently by different cultures, the Romans used it medicinally, ancient Egyptians called it Tham and used the plant in embalming. The Greeks knew of two type, Dioscorides talked of white- for medicinal purposes and the black was not favored as it ' corrupted the organism and provoked the secretion of bile. It is well known for its digestive properties.

Emotional : During eighteenth century it was recommended for nervous disorders as it strengthens nervous system and reestablish strength in convalescence.

Digestive : Digestive properties of Thyme were known since olden times as infusions of the herb were consumed at the end of banquets for digestive purposes. It is a tonic, stimulant, stomachic and digestive : relieves gastritis enterocolitis and mouth thrush.

Respiratory : It is a useful oil for respiratory infections, asthma and bronchitis.

Muscular : Thyme is effective for treating swellings provoked by gout or rheumatic problems, for joint pains, backache and sciatica.

Gynecological: Thyme Oil is useful for urinary and vaginal infections, endometritis (candida), prostates, and vaginitis, can be used in douche or sitz bath.

Caution: *May cause skin irritation in sensitive people.*

Essential Oil of Vertiver

(Vertiveria zizanoides-Gramineae/ Poaceae)

Vertiver grass is cultivated in tropical and sub tropical climates. The grass, is a close relative of other aromatic grasses such as lemon grass, is upright with narrow odourless leaves, it is the roots that have a strong scent, similar to sandalwood or violets. In India, Vertiver is known as Khus. The grass has to be at least two years old before the roots can be dried in the hot sun.

Part of the plant used: Root

Method of extraction: Steam Distillation

Volatility: Base note

Principal constituent: An alcohol called Vertiverol, vertiveryl acetate.

Properties, effects and method of use

The oil is dark brown with a warm peppery, spicy, woody earthy smell, Known as the oil of tranquility, vertiver imparts a sense of calm and peacefulness. It is therefore ideal in the times of stress, tension and physical or mental exhaustion. In beauty care, the oil enables the skin to retain water more readily, making it one of nature's best moisturisers.

Emotional- Calming and relaxing, beneficial for relieving stress, tension, physical or mental exhaustion, especially effective in post partum depression. Used in inhalations, vaporizer baths, application or massage.

Skin- Soothing and moisturizing, vertivert plumps out the tissues of the skin and helps to bring back a more youthful softness to mature skin.

Digestive : The oil helps clear liver congestion.

Gynecological: The oil is female tonic and hormone regulator, relieves amenorrhoea.

Aromatherapy applications- Bath (p.m.), Facial Care, Hand Care, Massage oil for hard, dry, wrinkled / aging skin and also for breast development.

Caution-*Beware of adulterated oils with synthetics as the adulterated versions have noxious effect on the skin.*

Essential Oil of Wintergreen

(Gaultheria procumbens-Eriaceae)

The leaves of evergreen flowering shrub, native of United States and Canada, also found in mountainous areas of Indian sub continent. In America, it also called partridge berry or checkerberry and has been used by Indians for its remarkable therapeutic properties. They masticated the leaves when they had pain or fever, prepared refreshing drinks with them and also fed the barriers to their animals.

The leaves of the plant have to have to be macerated for up to 24 hours in hot water in order to produce the fermentation which releases the essentials of the plant.

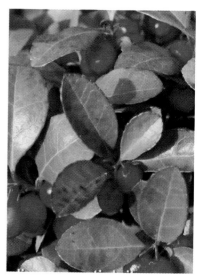

Part of the plant used: Leaves and berries.

Method Of Extraction: Maceration/ Distillation

Volatility : Top Note

Principal constituents: 90 to 95 % methyl salicylate, ketone, secondary alcohol and an ester.

Properties, effects and method of use:

Renowned for its anti rheumatic properties, the oil is colorless but when older becomes reddish brown, has a characteristic camphoraceous smell noticeable in most of the pain balms and liniments, however the synthetic version of oil-Methyl salicylate is used often for price consideration.

Emotional- Highly aromatic and reminiscent of camphor with a note of Vanillin, the aroma provides mental clarity, relieves mental fatigue, also helpful in headaches & migraines.

Respiratory- The strong aroma helps to clear nasal, sinus and bronchial congestions.

Muscular- The oil is renowned for its anti rheumatic properties and its beneficial effect on muscular system; it helps in gout and stiffness due to old age. Even the leaves of the plant can be warmed up applied as poultices for muscular and rheumatic swellings.

Circulatory- Wintergreen is having diuretic effect, helps circulation and decongestion of lymphatics, it can also be used in the treatment of cellulite in combination with other oils.

Gynecological- The oil is stimulant and emmenagogue, also relieves menstrual cramps.

Caution: Mostly Methyl salicylate is sold as Winter Green oil, so better check from your source. Methyl Salicylate, being a chemical may cause skin sensitization if applied directly.

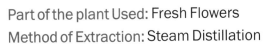

Essential Oil of Ylang Ylang

(Cananga odorata var. genuina)

Water or steam distillation of the flowers of the tall, tropical trees from Asia, commonly called Cananga. Most of the Ylang Ylang is produced in Madagascar, Phillipines, reunion, and the Comoros Island. There are four grades of Ylang Ylang 1,2,3 and also a Ylang Ylang extra, which is more expensive and have a superior Fragrance. The islanders used the oil on their body during rainy season to protect themselves from contagious illnesses and infections. Some use to mix the oil with coconut oil and apply on the hair before getting in the sea, to protect their hair.

Part of the plant Used: Fresh Flowers

Method of Extraction: Steam Distillation

Volatility: Middle Note

Principal Constituents: Alpha pinene, Sesqui-terpenes -cadinene, caryophyllene, benzoic acid, cresol, eugenol, 5-7% linalyl acetate, 8-10% linalyl benzoate, 30-32 % linalool and geraniol.

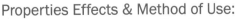

Properties Effects & Method of Use:

Ylang Ylang is a pale yellow liquid with an intensely sweet, floral scent reminiscent of a blend of jasmine and almonds. The oil has been found to be anti infectious and have a good result in Malaria, thypus and other fevers.

Emotional- Ylang Ylang is sedative, helps calm the nerves, good hypotensive, reduces palpitation, hypertension and high blood pressure. Its odor effect is intoxicating and antidepressant; a reputed aphrodisiac good support for fidgidity.

Skin & Hair- Ylang Ylang promotes hair growth, controls dandruff. It can be used in skin formulations to tan the skin (should avoid over exposure to sun).

Respiratory- The anti infectious properties of the oil help in respiratory and pulmonary infections.

Circulatory- The oil reduces hypernoea (over accelerated breathing rate) and tachycardia (abnormal rapidity of heart beat). It is a good hypotensive and helps reduce blood pressure.

Digestive- Ylang Ylang is an antispasmodic and antiseptic for intestinal infections, diarrhea and flatulence.

Gynecological- A balancer of female immune system it helps in PMS reduces negative emotions, tensions, cramps and headaches.

Caution: *The oil is extracted in many stages and so many fractions are taken out, all qualities are sold*

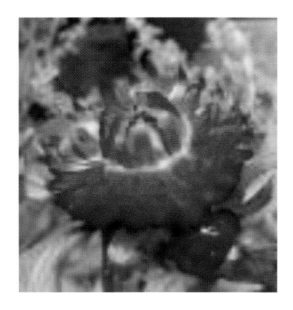

Helichrysm

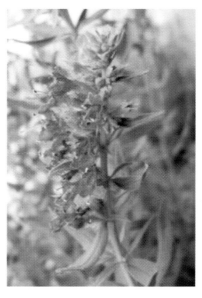

Hyssop

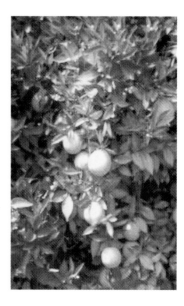

Orange

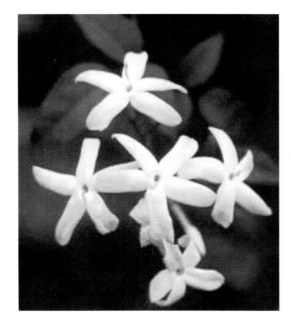

Jasmine

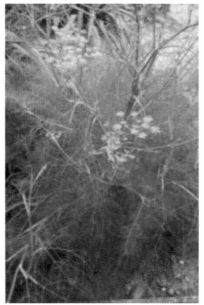

Fennel Sweet

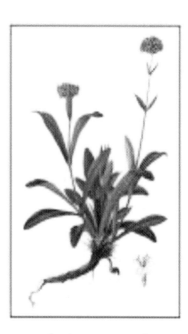

Jatamansi

Profiles of other important Essential Oils

Angelica

(Angelica archangelica)

Source: The essential oil is obtained by steam distillation of roots or the seed from the plant which is native to Europe and Siberia.

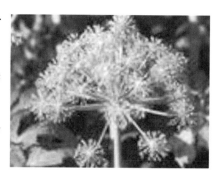

Principal Constituents: Angelicin, bergaptene, phellandrenic compounds and other terpenes.

Aromatherapy uses: Psoriasis, arthritis rheumatism, respiratory ailments, fatigue, nervous tension, cold and flu.

Description and odour effect: The root oil is colorless, turning yellow and then dark yellow as it ages. It has a rich herbaceous-earthy scent. The seed oil is colorless and has a fresher, spicy top note. The odor effect of both oils is stimulating and aphrodisiac.

Caution: *The root oil (not seed oil) should not be applied to the skin shortly before exposure to sunlight as it may cause pigmentation, Avoid during pregnancy.*

Aniseed/Anise

(Pimpinella-Anisum)

Source: The essential oil is distilled from the seed fruits of a tender annual plant from orient also known as sweet cumin.

Principal constituents: Anethole 80 to 90% with little aldehyde, anisic Acid and methyl Chavicol.

Aromatherapy Uses: The main property of anise is digestive, in premenstrual tension and menopausal symptoms. Used mostly as tisane, it helps indigestion due to anxiety and nervousness, relaxation after meal.

Description and odour effect: The oil is colorless or very pale yellow, smells very sweet and very characteristic, a little like fennel.

Caution: *The essential oil is very toxic and dangerous - a real poison for the nervous system may cause muscular numbness followed by paralysis.*

Bergamot

(Citrus bergamia)

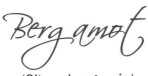

Source: *Obtained by expression of the rind of the small orange-like fruit native to Italy.*

Principal Constituents: *Upto 50% linalyl acetate, bergamotine, bergaptene, d-limonene and linalool.*

Aromatherapy uses: *Colds and flu, fever, infectious illness, tonsillitis (a few drops in water to be used as gargle), anxiety, depression.*

Description and odour effect: *A light green essence with a delightfully citrus aroma with a hint of spice. Refreshing and uplifting to the emotions.*

Caution: *Not to be used on the skin shortly before exposure to sunlight as it may cause pigmentation. However, for skin application try to obtain rectified bergamot oil called 'Bergamot FCF', which is free of bergaptene (the substance which causes skin pigmentation). However, whole bergamot oil can be used as a room scent.*

Benzoin

(Styrax benzoin)

Source: *Steam distillation of the gum resin exudes from the bark of the tree native of Laos and Vietnam but now grows in and around Malaysia, Java and Sumatra.*

Aromatherapy uses: *Skin care (particularly for eczema and psoriasis), frostbite, bedsores, wounds and skin ulcerations, also useful for catarrh and chest infections.*

Description and odour effect: *A colorless to Pale yellow liquid with strong vanilla like fragrance.*

Principal Constituents: *20-25% Cinnamic acid, vanillin, coniferyl benzoa te, benzoic acid, phenylethylene and phenylpropylic alcohol.*

Black Pepper

(Piper nigrum)

Source: Steam distillation of the dried peppercorns from a woody vine native to South west India. Most of the oil is produced in India, although it is also distilled in Europe and the USA from the imported peppercorns.

Principal Constituents : Monoterpenes (4%), Sesquiterpenes 985-90%) few alcohols, ethers, ketones, aldehydes, acids and a nitrogen compound N femyryl.

Aromatherapy uses: Poor circulation, muscular aches and pains, loss of appetite, nausea, colds and flu, infections and viruses, lethargy, mental fatigue.

Description and odour effect: A pale, greenish-yellow liquid with a hot, spicy, piquant odour. The smell is stimulating and warming; a reputed aphrodisiac.

Caution: Use in low concentration; avoid on sensitive skin.

Cade

(Juniperus oxycedrus)

Source: Steam distillation of the young twigs and wood from Mediterranean equivalent of the common Juniper.

Principal constituents: Phenol (Creosol guaiacol), Sesquiterpenes (Cadiene) and other terpenes.

Aromatherapy Uses: Pure oil is one of the best remedies for hair loss, dandruff, hair weakened by dyeing and bleaching and skin eruptions.

Description and odour effect: The oil is resinous, darkish brown colour, and as a strange waxy smell that is even caustic and tarlike.

Caution: Cade is often adulterated with pine, birch petrol and tar, so be sure of the quality, adulterated oil can provoke terrible skin reactions.

Cajeput

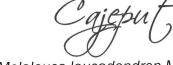

(Melaleuca leucadendron-Myrtaceae)

Source: Cajeput name is derived from Malay *"kayu-puti or caju-puti"* meaning white trees, from a variety of species from the same family of Tea tree and Niauli. It is the young twigs, leaves and buds which are fermented before distillation.

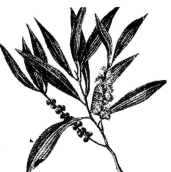

Principal Constituents: Cineol (40-70%), pinene and terpineol along with aldehydes like benzoic, butyric, valeric.

Aromatherapy Uses: Useful oil for rheumatism and stiff joints also a valuable treatment for cystitis. Can also be used for bursitis, chest infections, colds, cough, hay fever, headaches, sore throat etc.

Description & Odour Effect: Oil is colorless to pale with camphoraceous, spicy aroma helps clear nasal congestion and headaches.

Caution: The should not be used internally.

Camphor Borneol

(Dryobalanops Aromatic/ Camphora)

Source: Steam distillation of evergreen plant native to the west coast of Sumatara and the north of Borneo.

Principal Constituents: Main constituent is terpinic alcohol- Boroneol

Aromatherapy Uses: Borneol camphor is one valued in Ayurvedic system of medicine, for many centuries, it is used in combination with other plants for eye injuries, infections, headaches and migraines. Considered good for insect and snake bites, inflammations, muscular and rheumatic pain, cuts and bruises. It is renowned as tonic for the kidneys as adiuretic and strong antiseptic helps in leucorrhea and vaginitis.

Description: Smells primarily of Camphor, the oil is pale yellow and does not crystallize easily. It is only the borneol in the oil, which crystallizes in small grains or thin layers oil.

Caution: Do not use Camphor with homeopathic medicines it will affect their efficacy.

Camphor Wood

(Cinnamomum Camphora)

Source: Steam distillation of clippings, wood and root of an evergreen tree native to China, Taiwan and Japan. Older the tree, more the oil it contains.

Principal Constituents: Main constituents include azulene, Boroneol, Cadinene Camphene, Carvacrol, Cineol, Cuminic alcohol, Dipentene, eugenol, phellandrene, pinene, Sajrol and terpineol.

Aromatherapy Uses: Oil is good for inflammations, muscular and rheumatic pain, cuts and bruises also used as an insect repellant.

Description: Crystalline ketone camphor $(C10H16)$ or Solid Camphor and its pale yellow oil is extracted from old plants.

Cardamom

(Elettaria cardamomum)

Source: Steam distillation of the dried ripe fruit (seeds) from the reed-like herb native to Asia.

Principal Constituents: Cineol and terpineol, with a little limonene.

Aromatherapy uses: Digestive disturbances, mental fatigue, nervous exhaustion.

Description and odour effect: A colourless to yellowish liquid with a sweet-spicy, warming fragrance. The odor effect is warming and stimulating; a reputed aphrodisiac,

Caution: Use in the lowest concentration as it has a high odor intensity.

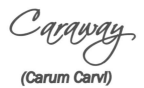

Caraway

(Carum Carvi)

Source: *Steam distillation from plant native to south eastern Europe.*

Principal constituents: *50 to 60% carvone, others are carvacol, carvene and limonene. Research has confirmed that high percentage of carvone help in digestion stimulation and release of gastric juices.*

Aromatherapy uses: *Caraway is excellent for all digestive problems like flatulence, pain, dyspepsia Cclic and colitis. The oil is also considered to be a mild antiseptic an effective remedy for Vertigo.*

Description and odour effect: *The oil is sometimes with a tinge of yellow, which darkens as the oil matures. The smell is muskier than cumin, more fruity and hot.*

Caution: *Due to high ketone contents the oil should be used with caution.*

Celery

(Apium graveolens- umbelliferae)

Source: From hardy biennial vegetable grown for its crisp, long crescent shaped stalks, though oil can be extracted from all parts but the oil from seeds is preferred for therapeutic use.

Principal Constituents: Lactone sedanolide, palminic acid and terpinic hydrocarbons- limonene and selinene.

Aromatherapy Uses: Hippocrates and Dioscorides thought of it as a strong diuretic also used for chilblains. It can be used as raw or cooked vegetable also, particularly good for diabetics, who suffer from hypoglycemia. It is also considered to be a good aphrodisiac. Celery juice helps in cystitis besides helping in menstrual complaints.

Description & Odour Effect: The Celery seed oil is pale yellow liquid with strong celery aroma.

Cinnamon Bark

(Cinnamonum zeylanicum)

Source: Steam distillation of the bark chips from the small tree native to Sri Lanka, India and Madagascar. A low grade oil is obtained from the leaves and twigs.

Principal Constituents: Cinnamic aldehyde (60-70 %) caryophllene, cymene, eugenol, linalol, pinene etc.

Aromatherapy uses: Cinnamon is highly microbial, used in the vaporizer as an antiviral fumigant during infectious illness also useful as antidepressant room scent or as an antibiotic. Taken as a tisane Cinnamon is good for circulation, detoxifies and helps burn fat.

Description and odour effect: A light amber liquid with a sweet, warm-spicy, dry, tenacious aroma. The odour effect is stimulating and warming; a reputed aphrodisiac.

Caution: This oil is a powerful skin irritant. Use only as a room scent.

Clove Bud

(E_ugenia caryophyllus)

Source: Water distillation from the buds of the slender evergreen tree native to Indonesia. Most supplies of the oil are from Madagascar. Lower grade of clove oil are distilled from the leaves and stems.

Principal Constituents: Phenols (70-80%) particularly Eugenol, acetyl eugenol, benzoic acid, benzyl benzoate and furfurol.

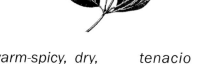

Aromatherapy uses: It is also employed as a first aid measure for toothache (the oil is analgesic), but should never be used in long-term as it is a skin irritant and will damage the gums. Whilst awaiting dental treatment, a single drop of the oil can be dropped into the tooth cavity or rubbed into the gums. Oil can be vaporized as a room scent, or used as a fumigant during infectious illness.

Description and odour effect: A light amber liquid with a bitter sweet spicy aroma. The odor effect is warming and stimulating. A reputed aphrodisiac.

Caution: The oil is a powerful skin irritant, so use only as a room scent. Use in the lowest concentration as it has a high odour intensity.

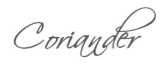

Coriander

(Coriandrum sativum)

Source: Steam distillation of the herb native to Europe and western Asia. Most of the oil is produced in Eastern Europe.

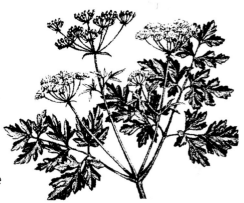

Principal Constituents: An alcohol (coriandrol, 60-65%), geraniol and pinene.

Aromatherapy uses: Arthritis, muscular aches and pains, poor circulation, digestive problems, colds and flu, mental fatigue and nervous exhaustion.

Description and odour effect: A color less to pale yellow liquid with a sweet, spicy, faintly musky aroma. It has a stimulating, warming aroma and is a reputed aphrodisiac.

Dill

(Anethum Graveolens)

Source: Steam distillation of the seeds of this plant of umbelliferae family.

Principal constituents: Oil in having high ketones contents mostly dextro-carvone and phenolic ethers.

Aromatherapy Uses: Dill seed oil is used in babies gripe water. It helps the flow of bile, thus aiding digestion, and is useful for catarrhal conditions like bronchus.

Caution: Because of high ketone contents the oil should not be used on children or pregnant women.

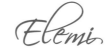

Elemi

(Canarium luzonicum)

Source: Steam distillation of the gum exudes from the tall tree native to the Philippines and the Moluccas.

Principal Constituents: Phellandrene, dispentene, limonene and pinene.

Aromatherapy uses: Rheumatic conditions, respiratory disorders, skin infections, nervous exhaustion.

Description and odour effect: A pale yellow or colourless liquid with a strong, spicy balasmic aroma which also has citrus-geranium note. The odour effect is tenacious, stimulating and warming.

Caution: *Use in the lowest concentration as it has high odour intensity.*

Fennel - Sweet

(Foeniculam vulgare)

Source: Steam distillation of the crushed seeds from the herb native to the Mediterranean region. Most of the oil is produced in Hungary, Bulgaria, Germany, France, Italy and Greece.

Principal Constituents: Anethol upto 60%, anisic aldehyde, camphene, d-fenchone, dipentene.

Aromatherapy uses: Bruises, cellulite, fluid retention, constipation, loss of appetite, flatulence, insufficient milk in nursing mothers, menopausal problems.

Description and odour effect: A colorless to pale yellow liquid with a sweet anise-like aroma. The odour effect is warming and stimulating.

Caution: *The oil may irritate the skin should be used with caution. Avoid during pregnancy. The oil has an intense odor, so use in small quantities.*
There is also a remote chance that fennel will promote an epileptic seizure, but only in prone subjects. Therefore, avoid if you suffer from epilepsy.

Galbanum

(Ferula galbaniflua)

Source: Water or steam distillation of the gum exudes of the large herb native to the Middle East and western Asia.

Principal Constituents: 50-60% Carvone, sesquiterpenes, sesquiterpenic alcohol (cadinol) and terpenes (limonene and pinene)

Aromatherapy uses: Abscesses, acne, scars, wounds, inflamed skin, poor circulation, muscular aches and pains, rheumatism, respiratory ailments, nervous tension and stress-related disorders.

Description and odour effect: An amber colored liquid, becoming viscous as it ages, with a green-woody scent and soft balsamic undertone. The odor effect is calming; a reputed aphrodisiac.

Caution: *Not to be used during pregnancy. The oil has an intense odor, so use in low concentration.*

Ginger

(Zingiber officinale)

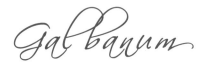

Source: Steam distillation of the unpeeled, dried, ground root (rhizomes) of the plant native to Southern Asia.

Principal Constituents: Sesquiterpenes (camphene, d-phellandrene, zingiberene), sesquiterpenic alcohols (isoborneol-linalool), and terpenes.

Aromatherapy uses: Arthritis, muscular aches and pains, poor circulation, rheumatism, catarrh, coughs, sore throats, diarrhea, colic, indigestion, nausea, travel sickness, colds and flu, debility, nervous exhaustion.

Description and odour effect: A pale yellow or amber liquid with a warm, peppery spicy scent, not as pleasantly pungent as the fresh root. Its odour effect is warming and stimulating; a reputed aphrodisiac.

Caution: *Use in minute quantities as the intense aroma - may overpower your blends.*

Grapefruit

(Citrus paradisi)

Source: Expression of the fresh peel of the fruit from a small evergreen tree native to tropical Asia. A low grade oil with a less attractive odour is obtained by steam distillation of the peel and fruit pulp. The oil is mainly produced in California.

Principal Constituents: Monoterpenes- limonene (96-98%), aldehydes, coumarins, flurocoumarins.

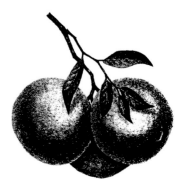

Aromatherapy uses: Cellulite, muscle fatigue, fluid retention chills, colds and flu, depression, nervous exhaustion.

Description and odour effect: The expressed oil (not the lower grade extraction) is a yellow-green liquid with a fresh, sweet citrus fragrance. Its odor effect is uplifting and anti-depressant.

Caution: *Do not apply to the skin shortly before exposure to sunlight as it may cause pigmentation.*

Helichrysm - Immortelle

(Helichrysm italicum/ H. angustifolia)

Source : One of the rare oils today, it is extracted by Steam distillation of flowers from Asteraceae or copmositae family.

Principal constituents : Sesquiterpenes mainly B caryophyllene, Monoterpenol- Nerol, Esters- Neryl acetate (75%) and Ketones B diones (Italidione I,II,III) up to 20 %

Aromatherapy Uses: Immortelle or Helichrysm was one of the oils used by Jesus for healing work. European researchers found Helichrysm as effective regenerator of tissues, nerves and circulation. Oil is useful for all skin problems like acne, infections, burns, eczema, bruising, cuts and dermatitis. Also useful for circulatory system, acts as detoxifier, decongestant and cleanser.

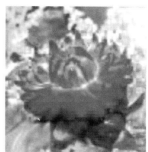

Description & Odour Effect: The oil has soft pervading sweet but uplifting aroma, helps to relieve anxiety, lethargy, tension, stress and shock.

Caution: *The oil may be neuro sensitive due to high ketone contents.*

Hyssop

(Hysoppus officinialis)

Source: Steam distillation of flower of hardy green busy plant with narrow dark leaves similar to those of lavender and rosemary.

Principal constituents: Alcohol, Gerniol, borneol, thujone, phellandrene, and in large quantities a terpenic Ketone - pinocamphone.

Aromatherapy Uses: Hyssop is pectoral, expectorant, decongestant, stimulant, sudorific and it is carminative. It is useful for coughs, flu, bronchitis, asthma and chronic catarrh. Hyssop can also be used externally and one of the recommendations is to use as a poultice of young bruised leaves on a bruise, cut or wound.

Description and odour effect: The plant is cultivated for its essential oil in different parts of France. This oil has very aromatic pleasant odour and is dark yellowish.

Caution: *The oil is potential neuro toxic because of pinocamphone it should be used with extreme Care or sold to health practitioners only or under a prescription.*

Jasmine

(Jasmine officinale)

Source: Jasmine is solvent extracted from two varieties of flowers named as Jasmine grandiflora (Chameli) and Jasmine sambac (Mogra) both are night-scented flowers from the evergreen climber native to China, northern India and western Asia. Most of the oil is produced in Egypt and France. In India both flowers are used to be worn as Veni (String) in the hair by women lending the senual smell to the hair.

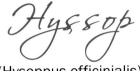

Principal Constituents: Mainly Jasmone, alpha terpineol, benzyl alcohol, indol, linalool and linalylacetate.

Aromatherapy uses: Reputed anti depressant and aphrodisiac, also good for nervous exhaustion and stress-related conditions.

Description and odour effect: The absolute is dark amber and slightly viscous with a warm, floral scent and musky undertone. The fragrance improves as the oil ages. The odor of Jasmine grandiflora is pervading sweet, sensuous but uplifting, while the fragrance of Jasmine sambac is highly uplifting with a citrus touch.

Caution: *The oil can be neuro sensitive due to high ketone contents*

Jatamansi (Indian Spikenard)

(Nardostachys jatamansi)

Source: Jatamansi is distilled from roots of a plant from India, of Valerianaceae family.

Principal Constituents: Sesquiterpenes (93%), isobornyl valerianate, bornyl acetate, pinene, terpineol, eugenol, borneol etc.

Aromatherapy uses: Reputed and regarded as a medicinal herb in India. It is antibacterial, antifungal and anti inflammatory. Helps in the treatment of skin allergies, rashes, candida, flatulence, tension, migraine, and insomnia.

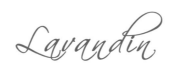

Description and odour effect: The oil is amber coloured having sedating effect on nervous system, helps in insomnia, nervous tension and migraines.

Caution: *Due to high citral contents the oil may sometimes, cause skin irritation in people with sensitive skin.*

Lavandin

(Lavendula fragrans/hybrida)

Source: Steam distillation of hybrid lavander, a cross between lavender and aspic.

Principal Constituents: Borneol (40 to 50%), Camphor (10%), Cineol(10%), Geraniol, Linalool and Linayl acetate (15 to 35%).

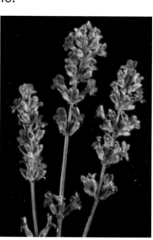

Aromatherapy Uses: The oil is mostly used in perfumery, but, it also good for muscular, respiratory and circulatory problems because of its high camphor contents.

Description and odour effect: Oil is yellow to dark yellow and smells acridly aromatic and little camphoric.

Caution: *Lavendin is less therapeutic than lavender but often sold as lavender.*

Lime

(Citrus aurantifolia)

Source: Expression of the peel of the unripe fruit of the small evergreen tree native to southern Asia. There is also a distilled oil which is captured from the whole ripe crushed fruit. Most of the oil is produced in Florida, Cuba, Mexico and Italy.

Aromatherapy uses: Cellulite, poor circulation, respiratory disorders, colds and flu, depression.

Description and odour effect: A pale yellow or green liquid with a fresh, citrus aroma. Try to use within one year of purchase as the aroma rapidly deteriorates with age. The odour effect is uplifting and refreshing.

Caution: *The expressed oil can cause unsightly blotching of the skin if applied shortly before exposure to sunlight, but the distilled oil is benign in this respect. However, the aroma of the expressed oil is superior.*

Lemon Grass

(Cymbopogan citratusi/flexuous)

Source: Steam distillation of leaves of tropical grass native of tropical asia and cultivated in India, Sri Lanka, Indonesia, Africa, Madagasscar, S & N America. Grass resembles closely to Palmarosa and citronella (under the same generic name Andropogan).

Principal constituents: Citral (70-85%), dispentene, citronellal, farnesol, geraniol, limonene, linalool, methyl leptanol, myrecene, n-decyclic aldeyde, nerol.

Aromatherapy Uses: Very good antiseptic and detoxifying agent, helps reducing temperature.

Description and odour effect: A pale yellow liquid with citrus top note, very good anti depressant and uplifting.

Caution: *Due to high citral contents the oil may sometimes, cause skin irritation in people with sensitive skin.*

Mandarin

(Citrus reticulate)

Source: Expression of the peel of the fruit of the small evergreen tree native to southern China and the Far East. Most of the oil is produced in Italy, Spain, Cyprus and Greece.

Principal constituents: Methylanthranilate, linionine, geraniol and terpenic aldehydes.

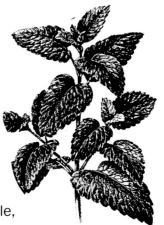

Aromatherapy uses: Relaxing and uplifting oil helps stretch marks, cellulite, fluid retention, digestive problems, insomnia, nervous tension.

Description and odour effect: A yellow - orange liquid with an intensely sweet citrus aroma. Try to use within one year of purchase as the aroma rapidly deteriorates with age. Its odor effect is soothing and uplifting.

Caution: *Do not apply to the skin shortly before exposure to sunlight as it may cause pigmentation.*

Melissa

(Melissa officinalis)

Source: Steam distillation of leaves and tops of hardy herbaceous perennial native to Southern Europe.

Principal constituents: Citral, citronellal, geraniol, linonene, linalool and pinene.

Aromatherapy uses: Melissa is a good anti depressant as per the clinical trials, besides being antispasmodic, an emmanagogic, stimulant for nervous system and tonic for cardiac system, good for headaches, anxiety, palpitation and insomnia.

Description and odour effect: Oil is pale yellow with an agreeable and subtle, warm, lemony aroma which is pleasantly uplifting.

Myrrh

(Commiphora myrrha)

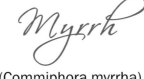

Source: Steam distillation of the gum of the small tree native to North-east Africa and South-west Asia. A solvent- extracted resinoid is also available, but this is not recommended for home use as it is solid at room temperature and therefore difficult to use.

Principal constituents: Acids (acetic, formic, myrrholic, palmitic, triterpenic etc.), alcohols, aldehydes (cinnamic, cuminic etc.), sugars (arabinose, galactose etc.), phenols (eugenol, m-creso), resins and terpenes (cadinene, dipentene, limonene, pinene etc).

Aromatherapy Uses: Athlete's foot, skin care (especially mature skins), ringworm, wounds, arthritis, respiratory disorders, gum infections, mouth ulcers, absence of menstruation outside pregnancy, thrush, nervous tension.

Description and odour effects: The essential oil is a light amber viscous liquid with a warm, balsamic odor which improves as the oil ages. Its odor effect is warming and relaxing.

Caution: *Not to be used during pregnancy.*

Myrtle

(Myrtus communis)

Source: Steam distillation of the fresh leaves of evergreen shrub originated in Africa and grows all around Mediterranean.

Principal Constituents: Oil contains lot of tannin, camphene, cineol, geraniol, linalool, pinene and myrtenol.

Aromatherapy uses: Oil is tonic, astringent, used in skin preparations. Also effective, against hemorrhoids, due to high tannic contents.

Description and odour effects: The oil is clear yellow to greenish yellow. It smells camphory and peppery green, rather like bay.

Niaouli

(Melaleuca viridiflora)

Source: Steam distillation of fresh leaves & twigs of evergreen tree growing principally in New Caledonia and Australia.

Principal constituents: Eucalyptol (50 % to 60 %) plus a few esters (butyric and isovalerianic), limonene, pinene and terpineol.

Aromatherapy uses: Strong antiseptic, prescribed mainly for Urinary system (cystitis and leucorrhea) and pulmonary trouble (bronchitis, catarrh, runny or stuffy nose).

Description and odour effect: Oil is pale yellow that can become dark yellow (depending on the copper content of the soil). It has strong hot smell, very balsamic with a note of camphor. It is similar to cajeput in aroma and therapeutic properties).

Nutmeg

(Myristica Fragrans)

Source: Trees that produce both nutmeg and mace are large evergreen native to the Moluccas. Nutmeg oil is steam distilled from nuts, crushed to a butter, oil imported from the islands, is redistilled in France to improve the quality. Mace is steam distilled from the arils.

Principal Constituents: Both oils contain myristicine, with small quantities of borneol, comphene, Cymol, dipentene, gltiraniol, linalool, pinene, sapol and terpineol and acetic, butyric, caprific formic and myristic acids.

Aromatherapy uses: In Eighteenth Century, in France, mace was classified as a Tonic and stimulant, as an aid for general fatigue, and as a brain stimulant. It is also revered for its digestive properties, for people who cannot assimilate food, for wind and premenstrual pain. Nutmeg too is a tonic, good for the heart and for convalescence. Nutmeg also has a reputation as an abortifacient.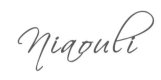

Description and odour effect: Both oils are similar, very pale yellow and very fluid. Nutmeg smells spicy, pleasant and hot, mace very strongly spicy. Both oils change as they become old, turning dark brown and smelling disagreeable acidic and turpentine like, hence should not be used.

Caution: *Myristicine is narcotic, hallucinogenic and very toxic especially during pregnancy. Nutmeg Mace oil should be avoided or used with great caution. It is better to use spice instead of oil for its therapeutic benefits.*

Orange sweet

(Citrus sinensis)

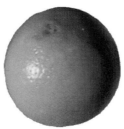

Source: Expression of the fresh ripe peel of the fruit of the small evergreen tree native to the Far East. An inferior grade steam distilled oil, obtained from the fruit pulp, is also available. Most of the oil is produced in Italy, Tunisia, Morocco and France.

Principal constituents: Upto 90% limonene with aldehydes, citral, citronellol, geraniol, linalool, methyl anthrinilate, nonyl alcohol and terpineol.

Aromatherapy uses: Palpitations, fluid retention, respiratory ailments, colds and flu, nervous tension, stress and depression.

Description and odour effect: A pale yellow liquid with a warm, sweet citrus scent. Try to use within one year of purchase as the aroma rapidly deteriorates with age. Its odor effect is uplifting.

Caution: *Do not apply to the skin shortly before exposure to sunlight as it may cause pigmentation.*

Oregano

(Oreganum Compactum)

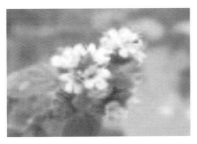

Source: Steam distilled from leaves and flowers of the plant from Labiatae (Mint) family mainly from Utah, Turkey and France.

Principal constituents: Monoterpnes (25%) alpha & Beta pinene, myrecene, sequiterpene, monoterpenols, linalool and phenols (60-72%), carvacrol, thymol.

Aromatherapy uses: Powerful anti infectious with large sectrum against bacteria, fungus and parasites for respiratory system, intestines, genitals, nerves, blood and lymphatics. The oil also helps in urinary infections, nephritis, digestive problems and balances metabolism. Can also be used on Skin warts.

Description and odour effect: An amber yellow liquid with a warm, pungent aroma, helps control fainting.

Petit grain

(Citrus aurantium var. amara)

Source: Steam distillation of the leaves and twigs of the bitter tree native to southern China and north-east India. Most of the oil is produced in France.

Principal constituents: Geraniol and geranyl acetate, limonene, linalool, linalyl acetate and sesquiterpene.

Aromatherapy uses: Oily skin conditions, nervous exhaustion and stress-related disorders.

Description and odour effect: A pale yellow liquid with a fresh, woody, bitter-sweet scent reminiscent of neroli, but less refined. Its odour effect is refreshing and uplifting.

Pine, Scotch

(Pinus sylvestris)

Source: Dry distillation of the needles of the evergreen tree native to Scotland and Norway.
Most of the oil is produced in the eastern USA from cultivated trees.

Principal constituents: Borneol acetate 30- 40 % (which is what differentiates it from turpentine) other terpenes are cadinene, dispentene and phedlandrene, pinene and sylvesterene.

Aromatherapy uses: Excessive perspiration, arthritis, muscular aches and pains, poor circulation, rheumatism, respiratory Ailments, cystitis, colds and flu, fatigue, nervous exhaustion.

Description and odour effect: A colorless to pale yellow liquid with dry-balsamic, turpentine-like aroma. Its odour effect is cooling, mentally stimulating, yet also comforting to the emotions.

Ravensara

(Ravensara aromatica)

Source: Steam distilled from the branches of a plantof Lauraceae family from Madagascar.

Principal constituents: Mono terpenes alpha & beta pinene, sesquiterpenes, monoterpenols, terpinic esters and oxides 1-8 cineol.

Aromatherapy uses: Excessive perspiration, arthritis, muscular aches and pains, poor circulation, rheumatism, respiratory Ailments, cystitis, colds and flu, fatigue, nervous exhaustion. Described as the oil that heals in Madagascar, it is found to be anti infectious, antibacterial, antiviral, antimicrobial and expectorant. It is tonic for nerves and respiratory system, effective for bronchitis and respiratory infections. Useful, in the treatment of herpes simplex and herpes zoster. Also helps in childhood viral infections like chicken pox and measles.

Description and odour effect: A colorless to pale yellow liquid helpful for fatigue, burnout and tensions.

Rosewood

(Aniba rosaeodora)

Source: Steam distilled from the wood of a plant of Lauraceae family, from Brazil.

Principal constituents: Monoterpenols mainly linalool (85-95 %), little oxides, monoterpenes and sequiterpenes.

Aromatherapy uses: Due to its high alcoholic percentage the oil is effective and safe for skin care, good for bacterial infections, urinary, bronchial, ENT and skin conditions like dermatitis

Description and odour effect: A pale yellow liquid with sweet wood aroma helps to relieve mental and physical exhaustion, relieves depression.

Sage

(Salvia officinalis)

Source: Steam distillation of the flowers and leaves of hardy, evergreen shrubs native to southern Europe.

Principal Constituents: Borneol, camphor, cineol, alpha pinene, salvene and Thujone (22 – 61%).

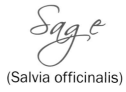

Aromatherapy uses: Sage has been cultivated for centuries for its culinary and medicinal properties. It helps in several skin conditions such as eczema, alopecia and ulcers. Helps in rheumatic and general aches and pains. Alleviates low blood pressure, purifies blood, regulates menstrual flow, a good diuretic and beneficial in Menopause.

Description and odour effect: The oil is colorless to pale yellow with strong herbaceous smell.

Caution: *Due to its Thujone content, oils can stimulate nervous system and can cause epileptic fits in prone subjects – Use with care.*

Savory

(Satureja horensis [summer]); (Satureja montana [winter])

Source: Steam distillation from the leaves (sometimes the flowers are also used) of two major Savory varieties, summer Savory – a bust annual a foot height with dark green aromatic leaves, hairy stems and pink-lilac flowers. Winter savory is compact and erect with small grey green leaves and tiny rose purple flowers. Both are plants of Mediterranean region.

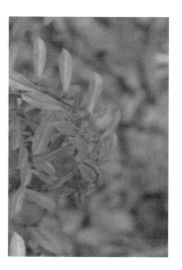

Principal constituents: The oil has very high phenol contents and other constituents are 30 to 40% carvacrol, 20 to 30% thymol and cineol, cymene and pinene.

Aromatherapy uses: Oil is strongly antiseptic because of high phenol contents, should be used in dilutions very useful for hastening the formation of scar tissue and for treating bites, burns, ulcers and abscesses. Herb tea with fresh savory is a great tonic and wine with savory is an aphrodisiac.

Description and odour effect: *The oil is Pale orange, quite hot, like thyme and a bit acrid.*

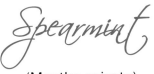

Spearmint

(Mentha spicata)

Source: Oil is produced by steam distillation of the leaves of evergreen plant of Lamiaceae family.

Principal constituents: Borneol Monoterpenes- limonene, pinene, myrecene etc along with monoterpenols- menthol, linalool, ketones (55-65%)- carvone, di hydro carvone and menthone.

Aromatherapy uses: Digestive oil good for acidity, heart burns, intestinal parasites and bad breath, also helps in hot flushes, nausea, nervousness, headaches and migraines.

Description and odour effect: A greenish yellow liquid with strong minty aroma commonly used for chewing gums, candies and toiletries.

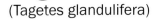

Tagets

(Tagetes glandulifera)

Source: Steam distillation of the flowers of the African Marigold plant, some times confused with calendula.

Aromatherapy uses: Effective on slow to heal wounds, burns and bruises, it is also useful against catarrhal conditions. Competent on fungal infections of the feet and of the digestive system (Candida), it may also promote the on set of menstruation. It is an excellent deterrent to house flies.

Principal constituents: Contains approximately 35-50% tagetone, a Ketone, and its coumarin content makes it a photo sensitizer.

Caution: *Being neuro- toxic it should be used in controlled manner. Not recommended for use on pregnant women or on children. Do not use immediately before exposure to sun.*

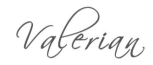

Valerian

(Valeriana officinalis/V.Wallichi [Indian Valerian])

Source: Steam distillation of the fresh well dried roots.

Principal constituents: The chemical constituent responsible for the aroma and therapeutic effect is bornyl-isovalerate, which develops as the roots are dried.

Aromatherapy uses: It is used almost exclusively for its powerfully calming effect on the nervous system, thus aiding all conditions related to severe mental stress e.g. insomnia, agitation, nervous headaches, nervouse stomach, palpitaions etc.

Description and odour effect: Used as the blue print for valium the well known sedative drug valerian is known in aromatherapy for its rather pungent aroma. The aroma of Indian Vallerian (V. Wallichi) is considered inferior; being strong the oil is yellowy brown in colour.

European Valerian oil (V. officinalis) is blue- green depending on the amount of azulene produced during distillation).

Caution: *Over use for along period may cause lethargy. Use only one drop in addition of petitgrain, orange or mandarin to improve the aroma.*

Carriers and Carrier Oils

A carrier is which carries. All essential oils applications require a carrier, not necessarily, an oil. We use various carriers, knowingly or unknowingly. Even in a simple process of inhalation the air acts a carrier, in bath, sitz bath, douche etc. its water which acts as a carrier. It's very rare that an essential oil is used undiluted. Only a few essential oils, can be used undiluted, since essential oils are highly concentrated and may sensitize the skin, if used neat. Therefore it is recommended that we dilute essential oils in fatty / vegetable oils also called base oils, before we use them on the skin, sometimes creams or lotions or gels are also used as carriers.

Carrier or base Oils-

Most preferred aromatherapy base or carrier oils for skin application are cold pressed vegetable oils. These vegetable oils contain essential fatty acids. They also penetrate easily, through the skin pores and provide nourishment, besides facilitating essential oils penetration in the body. The vegetable oils contain certain benefits themselves, not only for their contents of iodine, vitamin E and essential fatty acids (EFAs), they also act as balancing and stabilizing agent. The essential fatty acids are also needed by the body as a part of our regular dietary intake, also called vitamin F. We need to take in a variety of fatty acids, the most common ones are oleic acid, linoleic acid and linolenic acid.

The fatty acids are of two types, saturated fatty acids and unsaturated fatty acids. The oils rich in saturated fatty acids are generally too thick and greasy they are not preferred for aromatherapy use. The unsaturated fatty acids are classified into two groups- monounsaturated fatty acids and polyunsaturated fatty acids.

Oils with higher percentage of monounsaturated fatty acids (oleic acid), like almond, apricot, olive, hazelnut, camellia etc. are more stable and keep well for long time. The oils with higher percentage of polyunsaturated fatty acids (linoleic acid and linolenic acid) are light, not too greasy, but tend to break down easily therefore prone to oxidation. The oils rich in polyunsaturated fatty acids are good for heart but in aromatherapy, we need to choose a fatty oil, which will not oxidize too readily. Oxidized fatty oils have free radicals which are dangerous to the cells of the body. When a massage oil (consisting of essential oils in a fatty oil base) becomes rancid or oxidized, a chemical change takes place. This not only affects the fragrance of the blend and prevents the essential oils from working properly, but if massaged into the skin, can introduce cell damaging free radicals causing skin irritation. Therefore choosing a correct carrier or base oil is as important as choosing correct essential oils.

Carrier oils can be divided into three categories –

Basic oils – they form highest proportion (40-60%) of an aromatherapy formulation, since they are easily available or low in price etc. for eg. grapeseed oil, sesame seed oil, sunflower oil etc.

Specialized fixed oils- more often used as a certain percentage (10-30 %) of the main mix; perhaps too thick or expensive to be used on their own. They render specific therapeutic or nourishing and moisturizing property, to the whole mix for example Jajoba, Avacado, Wheatgerm, Evening Primrse, Hazelnut etc.

Macerated oils – are the plant extracts in a basic fixed oil. There are a few plants which contain very interesting properties, but whose essential oils are too difficult or too expensive to distil. In order to benefit from these properties, such oils are chopped up and put into a vat containing vegetable oil or water; this process is called maceration. The vegetable oil acts as a solvent, drawing essential oil from the plant material, including the small molecules as well as larger molecules such as plant coloring. The resulting liquid is then filtered and bottled. Macerated oils include Calendula, Carrot, Hypericum, Lime blossom and Melissa.

Those fatty oils consisting primarily of oleic acid are called mono- unsaturated oils (Mono meaning one) as this fatty acid has only one double bond in its chemistry. The higher the proportion of oleic acid the more stable the oil, it oxidizes much slowly than the fatty acids containing varying proportions oleic and other fatty acids. When a fatty oil contains a large amount of other fatty acids linoleic and linolenic, the oil is known as a poly-unsaturated oil (Poly meaning many) as these have two or three double bonds respectively. Please refer to the chart of fatty acids, listing the oleic, linoleic and linolenic acids in the vegetable oils. The chart should be used as a guide to choose the best oil for your formulations, as per the availability and limitation of your budget.

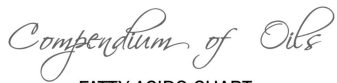

Compendium of Oils

FATTY ACIDS CHART

Oils		% Oleic	% Linoleic	% Linolenic	
Almond (Sweet)	M	70	20	—-	N
Apricot	M/P	65	27	—-	N
Avocado	M	70	9	—-	N
Camellia	M	78-92	1-2.2	—-	N
Coconut	Sat	6.5	1.5	—-	—
Corn	P	19-49	34-62	1-2.7	S
Cotton Seed	P	15.3-36	35-54.8	—-	S
Grapeseed	P	14	74	—-	S
Hazelnut	M	77	10	—-	N
Olive	M	65-85	3.9-15	0-1	N
Peach Kernel	M/P	68	25	—-	N
Peanut	M	42.3-61.1	13-33.4	—-	N
Pumpkin	P	35	45	—-	S
Rapeseed*	P	12-18	12-42	7-9	S
Rice	P	40-50	29-42	0-1	S
Rose hip seed	P	15	47	28-30	N
Safflower	P	13	75	—-	S
Sesame	M	35-46	35.2-48.4	0.2	N
Soya bean	P	32.5-30.8	49.2-52	1.9-10	D
Sunflower	P	33	52	0-1	S
Walnut	P	15	55	10-12	S

Jojoba - Liquid wax

Key
M – Mono-unsaturated
P – Poly-unsaturated
M/P – borderline between mono-saturated and poly - unsaturated
Sat – Saturated
N – Non - drying
S - Semi - drying
D - drying

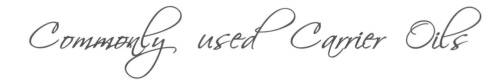

Commonly used Carrier Oils

Almond Oil, Sweet (Prunus amygdalis var. dulcis)-

The sweet almond tree yields a fixed oil obtained by cold pressing. There exists an essential oil from bitter almonds, should not be used in aromatherapy; because of the risk of prussic acid forming during distillation.

Properties and Effects: Sweet almond oil contains vitamins A, B1, B2 and B6 and has a high percentage of mono- and poly- unsaturated fatty acids. It has high percentage of mono-unsaturated fatty acids therefore keeps reasonably well. Because it has a small amount of vitamin E, it protects and nourishes the skin and calms the irritation caused by eczema.

Apricot Kernel Oil (Prunus armenica)-

Apricot, peach and sweet almond yield almost the same oils chemically (therefore having similar effects). Apricot and peach are usually more expensive as they are not produced in such great quantity. Occasionally almond oil is sold as apricot or peach, so be sure of the source of your oil.

Avocado Oil (Persea americana)-

Avocado oil is pressed from the dried and sliced flesh of fruits which are not good enough for marketing as fresh produce. Being quite a difficult oil to press, it sometimes has a cloudy appearance - even a bit sludgy at the bottom. This should be regarded as a good sign and not a fault.

Avocado oil has excellent keeping qualities because of an inbuilt antioxidant system, if chilled (or during the winter), some components are precipitated, causing it to go cloudy. This can be rectified by placing the bottle in a warm place, when the oil will soon return unharmed to normal.

Properties and Effects: Avocado contains both saturated and monounsaturated fatty acids and vitamins. (A, B and D) and is rich in lecithin, it is thought that despite its viscosity, avocado has the ability to penetrate the upper layers of the skin.

Avocado is valuable to the aromatherapists on account of its beneficial effect on dry skin and wrinkles, and it can form up to 25 per cent of the total mix. It is sometimes used for dry skin and in sun preparations on account of its emollient properties.

Calendula Oil (Calendula officinalis)- Macerated oil

Although sold as a fixed oil, the calendula grown in Europe for medical purpose does not produce any fixed oil itself. The flower-heads contain too little essential oil to make distillation commercially viable, so all active therapeutic properties are extracted by maceration.

Properties and Effects: Calendula oil has anti-inflammatory, anti-spasmodic, choleretic (increasing bile production) and vulnerary (helps in healing wounds) properties, rendering effective on bed sores, broken veins, bruises, gum inflammations (and tooth extraction cavities), persistent ulcers, stubborn wounds and varicose veins. It is extremely effective on skin problems, rashes, and in particular, chapped and cracked skin, which makes it an excellent base oil to use when treating dry eczema.

N.B: *Hypericum and calendula make an excellent synergistic mix to which essential oils can be added. Although extremely beneficial on its own, the effects are enhanced when essential oils for the condition being treated are added to it. If adding 25% or less to a basic carrier oil, the addition of the extra essential oils becomes more important.*

Camelia (Camellia japonica)-

Camelia oil, as its full name suggests, comes from Japan. It is extracted from the seeds of an evergreen tree from Theacae family, primarily cultivated on the islands of Izu and kyushu of Japan. Its Japanese name is tsubaki oil and is used in exclusive restaurants for cooking tempura-vegetables and prawns dipped in butter before quick frying as the oil is very stable at high temperature.

Properties and effects: The oil is virtually odorless with very good keeping quality; having long life span, very slow to oxidize as long as the bottle is kept well closed and out of sunlight. The oil is fairly thick but not so greasy with excellent skin penetrating ability. In beauty care the stability of camellia oil makes it, by far a very useful fatty oil for facial and body use, as the dangers of rancidity and resultant free radicals are negligible. The skin penetrating properties of camellia oil, enhance the speed at which diluted essential oil reach the deeper levels of the skin.

Carrot oil (Daucus carot)- Macerated Oil

True fixed oil of carrot is extracted by maceration of the finely chopped traditional orange carrot roots in a vegetable oil and is rich in beta- carotene. It is called to be 'true' fixed oil of carrot, because there is an oil used extensively in the cosmetic industry called "Carrot oil", that has never seen a carrot! The African marigold (tagets) is also rich in beta-carotene and this is sold as "carrot" oil such as soya or sunflower. It has similar properties to true carrot, but the oil is extremely concentrated, with a deeper color and is not suitable for aromatherapy treatments.

Properties and Effects: True carrot oil is rich in beta-carotene, vitamins B, C, D and E, and essential fatty acids.

Useful on burns, carrot oil is anti-inflammatory. It is known to be an effective rejuvenator, delaying the ageing process, with repeated use. It is therefore a useful, ingredient in skin creams or oils which are used every day.

Cautions: *There are no contra-indications to the use of carrot oil, but excessive ingestion of carrots themselves, or juice, can cause hyper-vitaminosis (the palms of the hands and soles of the feet become orange and the body skin dry and flaky, taking on an orangey, sun-tanned look). If these symptoms are ignored, the whole system becomes toxic, causing death in extreme cases.*

Castor Oil (Ricinus communis)

Castor oil comes from a tall, quick-growing, perennial woody shrub or small tree. Native to India but is now seen in many warm countries. It is often grown as an ornamental, but is also of value as a windbreak and shade tree. It bears seed profusely, and it is these that are pressed for the oil. This was known to the Greeks and Romans as purgative or laxative, which is still the major role of the oil today; lots of common laxatives contain a proportion of castor oil.

Properties and effects : *It has a very viscid consistency, is colorless, has a slight fragrance and is disagreeable to taste. The major constituents are palmitic and other fatty acids, ricinoleic acid and glycerine.*

The ancient Egyptians called the oil Kiki, using it as an unguent for skin rashes, and in embalming. It is still useful for numerous skin complaints, ranging from eczema to dryness of the skin. For very dry eczema, mix two tablespoons of castor oil with one tablespoon of almond oil and 2 drops of wheat germ oil and apply gently to the affected part. Because the oil is so viscid, it is good idea to mix with a light carrier oil to help its penetration.

Coconut Oil (Cocos nucifera)

Coconut oil does not occur naturally, the white flesh, when pressed yielding an odorous solid fat which contains therapeutic properties. To obtain coconut oil the fat is subjected to heat (as in hot extraction) and the top, liquid fraction removed. This is usually deodorized for use in both the food and cosmetic industries, as its natural odor is overpowering even with the addition of essential oils. Being a fractionated oil its use in aromatherapy, where we insist on everything being complete and whole must be questioned hence not recommended.

Properties and Effects: *Coconut oil is an emollient on hair and skin; is reputed to help filter the sun's rays; however, on some people it can cause rashes, perhaps because it is not a complete product.*

Corn Oil (Zee mays)

This oil produced exclusively by hot extraction (the corn germ containing very little oil) – though a very light oil, it is not one of the preferred oils for aromatherapy

Evening Primrose Oil (Oenothera biennis)

Rich in linoleic acid, a polyunsaturated fatty acid, and containing a small percentage of gamma linoleic acid (GLA- said to reduce blood cholesterol), evening primrose oil is extremely useful for the prevention of heart disease. These essential fatty acids are vital for cell and body function and cannot be made by the body itself.

Properties and Effects: Taken internally, evening primrose oil is said to be invaluable for reducing blood pressure, controlling arthritis, relieving eczema, helping schizophrenia, fibrocystic breast condition and PMS and decreasing hyperactivity in children. However, it has been found that the doses usually prescribed are probably too low to have a noticeable and lasting effect.

N.B: Used externally, the oil is helpful for eczema, dry, scaly skin and dandruff and accelerates wound healing. For details on health benefits of evening primrose oil refer to full chapter on evening primrose oil towards the end of the book.

Grape Seed Oil (Vitis vinifera)

Like corn oil, Grape seed oil is produced by hot extraction; it has only about 12 per cent of oil in the seeds. The oil can be 'rescued' after steam extraction (before passing through the refining process) but the extra labor and time involved increases the price substantially.

Properties and Effects: Grape seed oil contains a high percentage of linoleic acid and some vitamin E and is one of the few oils which are cholesterol free and easily digested. It is a gentle emollient, leaving the skin with a satin finish without feeling greasy, therefore preferred for use on oily skin.

Hazelnut Oil (Corylus avellana)

Both male and female flowers are present on each hazelnut tree, the nut yield an amber yellow oil, with a pleasant aroma and a slight flavor of marzipan.

Properties and Effects: Oleic acid (a monounsaturated fatty acid) is the principal constituent, with a small proportion of linoliec acid (polyunsaturated fatty acid) also being present.

Hazelnut oil is said to penetrate the top layer of the skin slightly, being beneficial for oily or combination skins and effective on acne. It stimulates the circulation and also has astringent properties. It may be more economical, to use it in conjunction with a less expensive base oil. However, when using it for skin disorders, it should be used alone as the base, with added essential oils.

Jojoba oil (Simmondsia chinensis)

Jojoba (pronounced 'hohoba') is not oil, but a liquid wax, coming from a desert shrub it is the only plant in the world to contain liquid wax which replaced sperm whale oil in the cosmetics industry when the whale became an endangered species. It is an environmental aid, as planting it saves arid land from becoming desert - plantations cover around 40,000 acres in the United States. It is also used, instead of beeswax, as an emulsifier in creams. Since Jajoba is very stable, having extremely good keeping qualities as it doesn't contain glycerides and very little fatty acids but contains 97 percent wax esters.

Properties and Effects: The chemical structure of Jajoba not only resembles sebum, but the later can dissolve in it, which makes it a useful oil for oily skin, specially in cases of acne. Jajoba inhibits the production of excess sebum by imparting a light coating of wax to the skin, thus fooling the body into believing that enough sebum has been produced, it is this effect which makes Jajoba a natural choice for treating acne and dandruff. The fact that it also is indicated for dry scalp and skin, psoriasis and eczema, shows it to be a balancing oil. Jajoba contains an acid (myristic acid) which has anti-inflammatory properties, helpful when mixing a blend for rheumatism and arthritis. In hair care also no other oil can match the ability of Jajoba oil, to make hair look and feel healthy, as it forms a thin coating on the hair giving it strength and lusture.

Melissa Oil (Melissa officinalis)

Macerated Melissa oil is only produced in regions where Melissa is grown for distillation and tea production.

Properties and effects: Melissa oil is indicated for massage on 'heavy legs' (fluid retention), especially in combination with cypress essential oil. It is also beneficial on dry mature skins.

Olive Oil (Olea europaea)

Traditionally used for centuries in cooking and healing, virgin pressed olive oil is popular on supermarket shelves because of its monounsaturated fatty acid content, effective the prevention of high cholesterol and heart disease, as well as its wonderful flavor. Its green color is due to small percentage of chlorophyll in the flesh, from which the oil is taken; it is an ideal cooking oil for health conscious people.

Properties and Effects: Externally olive oil is emollient, soothing to inflamed skin and good for sprains and bruises. It is a little heavy for massage, but can be added 50/50 to a less viscous oil.

When ingested, it is not only prophylactic against heart disease, but is a help against hyperacidity and constipation.

Peach Kernel Oil (Prunus persia): See Apricot Kernel Oil.

Peanut Oil (Arachis hypogeae)

Peanut oil is less stable oil regarding keeping qualities and has quite a noticeable aroma (not unpleasant and not as strong as coconut). It is mostly available only in the refined state although a small quantity is cold pressed in France.

Properties and Effects: A hypoallergenic and emollient oil (particularly for arthritis and sunburn), peanut, rather oily to use on its own for massage, is perfectly acceptable for self-application to specific areas or to blend with another less viscous carrier oil.

Rose Hip Oil (Rosa cannia, R. mollis)

Coming mostly from wild plants, this oil is usually organic and yields, a lovely, golden red oil, often obtained, unfortunately, by solvent extraction.

Properties and effects: Research in Chile shows rose hip oil to be a tissue regenerator (perhaps due to its high unsaturated fatty acid content), making it an excellent oil for a mature skin. It has been shown to be effective on scars, wounds, burns (including sunburn), eczema and ageing.

Safflower Oil (Carthmus tinnctorious)

Safflower, like sunflower, belongs to the Compositae family and has an orangey yellow flower. Safflower seeds were discovered in 3,000-year-old Egyptian tombs and both flowers and seeds have been used in the past as dye.

Properties and Effects: Yet another oil, which is high in polyunsaturated fatty acids, safflower helps a number of circulatory problems and taken internally, it is said to be helpful for bronchial asthma. It is beneficial on painful, inflamed joints, sprains and bruises. It is one of the less stable oils (except when it is refined, when it has preservatives added to it).

Sesame Oil (Sesamum indicum)

The seeds of the sesame plant are contained inside a long nut and give a high yield of clear pale yellow oil when cold pressed.

Properties and Effect: The pressed oil is rich in vitamins and minerals, its vitamin E and sesamol content giving the oil excellent stability.

It is beneficial for dry skin, psoriasis and eczema and protects the skin to a certain extent, from the harmful rays of the sun.

Soya Bean Oil (Glycine soja)

Soya bean oil is usually obtained by solvent extraction, as the beans have low oil content. Prone to oxidation, it can be a sensitizer, so it may be wise not to use it in aromatherapy.

Sunflower Oil (Helianthus annus)

Although most sunflower oil is solvent extracted, we can obtain an oil from organically grown plants that is cold pressed. This oil has a lovely light texture and is very pleasant to use, leaving the skin with a satin-smooth, non-greasy feel.

Properties and Effect: Sunflower oil contains vitamins A, B, D and E (the principal one) and is high in unsaturated fatty acids, making it helpful against arteriosclerosis. It has a prophylactic effect on the skin and is beneficial to leg ulcers, bruises and skin diseases. Sunflower oil has diuretic properties, is expectorant and one of its constituents, inulin, is used in the treatment of asthma.

The leaves and flowers have been used in Russia for years against chest problems such as bronchitis.

Wheatgerm Oil (Triticum vulgare)

Wheat germ oil is of rich orangey brown color and due to its high vitamin 'E' content, is widely used to increase the keeping qualities of less stable oils - a minimum of 10 per cent should be added to the base oil, up to 20 per cent if the oil has low stability.

Properties and Effect: Wheat germ is useful on dry and mature skins though too heavy to use, by itself, for massage. Taken internally, it is said to help prevent varicose veins, eczema and indigestion and helps to remove cholesterol deposits from the arteries.

Caution: As it is from a protein, it could be contra-indicated for anyone prone to allergies.

Section-II

Aromatherapy Oils Blending.

Aromatherapy applications

Safety Guildelines

Using aromatherapy with other therapies

50 easy ways to use aromatherapy Essential oils

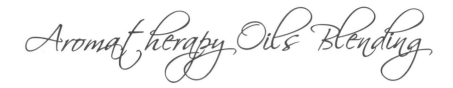

Pure essential oils are powerful, concentrated substances. They are normally used in very small quantity and diluted in a carrier oil or lotion, prior to use on the skin. This facilitates easy application, absorption and ensures against a skin reaction. For an aromatherapy formulation, we choose essential oils and carrier oils as per our specific requirement depending on client's assessment.

BLENDING

The art of blending aromatherapy oils depends on your ability to mix different complementary aromas to heal mind, body and the spirit.

Essential oils are synergists, complementing and enhancing each other's therapeutic actions. For this reason, blends of three to five essential oils are usually recommended for optimum therapeutic effect. To create your own blend, choose oils to suit your client's emotional and physical needs, favouring those, with aroma that appeal to everybody. Mix well and label clearly. Do not attempt to include more than five oils in a blend, since this may detract from their synergistic qualities.

RATIO or DOSAGE

The essential oils are used in small quantities almost 2 % in a blend; since it is difficult to measure very small quantity by weight / volume they are measured in terms of the number of drops. Depending upon the viscosity of the oil, one milliliter may contain 20 to 30 drops. So the easy way of calculating how much essential oil, to add, to a base oil is to measure the amount of base oil in milliliters and then add about half that number of drops of chosen essential oil.

For example:
* To a 50 ml bottle of base oil, add about 25 drops of essential oil - this gives approximately 2% -2.5% dilution. Add a few more drops for physical remedy, a few less for the treatment of sensitive or facial skin or an emotional or psychological problem.

*   To 1 tablespoon (approximately 15 ml) base oil add 6-9 drops of essential oil.

*   To 1 teaspoon (approximately 5 ml) carrier oil add 2-3 drops of essential oil.

SELECTING THE RIGHT ESSENTIAL OIL

Most important part of any therapy is "diagnosis" or assessing the cause of problem and choosing the right medicine for the condition, aromatherapy is no different. Essential oils are highly versatile in their therapeutic effect, meaning that a single oil may work for multiple conditions. For ease of choosing the right oils for blending, we first assess the conditions that need to be addressed. Then classify these conditions into –

<u>Primary</u>   <u>Secondary</u>   <u>Tertiary</u>

Now list all the essential oils options available to you, for each condition. Prepare a table format and from this table prefer the specialist oil suitable for each condition, needing maximum attention, prefer oils which are common for more than one condition. There by choosing, between three to five essential oils, for your blend. This way you cannot go wrong in your blends always keep in mind, if there is a caution associated for the use of any of the selected oil.
You can also choose your base or carrier oils the same way.

OIL BLENDING EQUIPMENTS

Besides the essential oils bottles being equipped with dropper plugs and a range of base oils you require the following to start with your essential oils blending.

1.   MEASURING CYLINDER: Measuring cylinders, cups and jars are available in various sizes from suppliers of laboratory equipments, if you are doing small quantities go for the small size cylinders say 100 Ml. with caliberations for each milliliter, for bigger batches you can go up to 500ml. Cylinders which may have caliberations for every 10 milliliters.

2.   STIRRING ROD : Glass stirring rods are required to stir the blends.

3.   STORAGE BOTTLES: Store the blended oils in dark coloured glass bottles.

4.   LABELS: All blends should be correctly labeled, try to incorporate a reference number and date of prepration.

5.   CLEANSING ALCOHOL : An alcohol like Iso-Propanol or rubbing alcohol is useful in cleaning your measuring cylinders and other equipments.

6.   CLEANSING TOWELS: All bottles, equipments and the table should be wiped after doing your blends. As the stickiness may spoil labels, attract dirt and make the place slippery and messy.

BASIC RULES OF BLENDING

There are certain basic rules to blending an aromatherapy formulation-

- Work out your quantities before you begin. First list all the essential and carrier oils required with dosages.

- Take out all the essential and base oils on the blending table.

- Check all the oils for caution / rancidity or oxidation. If you feel that there is a change in smell of the oil or if, the oil is looking turbid, do not use the same.

- Please ensure, that your measuring container, is clean, the best way to clean the measuring glass or cylinders is, with ethyl alcohol, ispo propyl alcohol or methanol and wiping it dry. All essential oils dissolve easily in the alcoholic solutions, even the residual base may also get dissolved in alcohol making these alcohols suitable for cleaning purposes. You can recycle this solvent at least few times before throwing it or better use it in a solution as a room scent/ freshener.

- Keep the clean bottles ready for filling the blended oil, label the same immediately after filling.

- Close all caps and plugs tightly.

- Wipe all the surfaces immediately and ensure there is spilled oil residue as the surface will get stained.

- Do not use or handle any plastic material, as neat essential oils react with plastics.

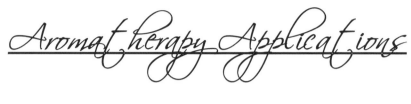

Aromatherapy Applications

Bath

Bath is the easiest and the most popular way of using essential oils. Few drops of Natural essential oils mix added to bath water improve body's immune level at physical level by penetration through skin pores, while the fragrance of the oil works at our mind (psychological level) by inhalation during the bath.

Simply add up to 5 drops in a bucket or up to 15 drops in the bath tub, of a chosen oil blend of pure essential oils. In case of shower bath, keep a mug full of water handy and add 5 drops essential oils, pour it over yourself once you finish the shower. Different essential oils can be selected for their specific effect - for example, lemongrass / rosemary are uplifting and stimulating, lavender/ geranium are soothing and relaxing, juniper berry helps in relieving fluid retention etc.

Essential oils can also be mixed in a teaspoon of vegetable oil (such as sweet almond oil) before adding to the bath. This helps to moisturize the skin and ensures an even distribution of the essential oils, which is important in the case of babies and young children. However, it may cause greasiness in the bathroom, making it slippery. Therefore it's advisable to use essential oils without base oils in the bath followed by a moisturizing blend.

To avoid possible irritation always check the safety data, before using, a new oil in the bath. Make up the few blends and keep them ready prepared. You can prepare the following two blends - uplifting blend will prepare you for the day ahead, while the relaxing blend is useful to relieve tension and restore harmony at the end of a stressful day.

Uplifting Bath Oil		Relaxing Bath Oil
3 ml of Lemon		3 ml of Lavender
2 ml of Basil		2 ml of Clary sage
2 ml of Juniper Berry		2 ml of Geranium
1 ml of Peppermint		1 ml of Patchauli
1 ml of Geranium		1 ml of Sandalwood

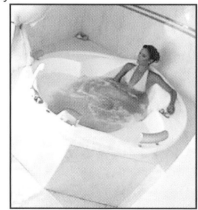

For each recipe, blend the essential oils in a brown-glass dropper bottle. Screw the bottle lids tightly shut, shake well, and label clearly.

Massage

Massage itself is a therapy in its own right, using essential oils add to the benefit of massage. According to Hippocrates it can "loosen a stiff joint" or "bind a loose joint". Therapeutic massage is the main method used by professional aromatherapists and also used in various SPA treatments for relaxation and detoxification. In aromatherapy massage the focus of the therapist should be on the movement and drainage of lymph. If it is not possible to carry out a full body massage, then a foot massage -using appropriate oils is an excellent alternative. When we massage the feet, we stimulate the rest of the body as well. This is because all the organs, glands and muscles in the human body have nerve ending located in the soles of the feet.

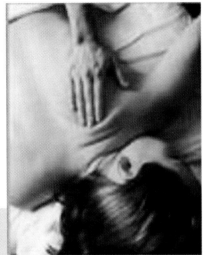

Massage works on us in multiple ways, not only it is a touch therapy which helps to soothe the mind and emotions, massage improves blood circulation resulting in to –

*More nutrients reaching skin surface and helping rejuvenation of the skin.

*Elimination of toxins at the fundamental level, helps to detoxify the body.

*Also helps to tone the body muscles.

PRIME FACTORS FOR MASSAGE-

Body massage is a well orchestrated movement of hands. Different parts of the world practice different kind of massage movement and techniques, however the popular types are Swedish massage, Shiatsu, Indian Ayurvedic massage, Thai Massage etc. Whatever type of massage you practice there are certain prime Factors which should be taken in to consideration.

1. **CONTACT-** When two energies come in contact initially there is a feeling of shock then they harmonize, therefore the contact, once established, should not be broken unless and until its necessary for eg. change of posture etc. In the process of massage if the contact is interrupted and re-established, there is a disturbance of energy that interferes in the relaxation of the client, which should be avoided.

2. **CONTINUITY-** Before starting the massage process all pending work including the visits to toilets should be taken care of, it is recommended to switch off the mobile (cell phones) too. As the process of massage once started should not be interrupted for any thing.

3. **PRESSURE-** Pressure is an integral part of massages. But each body type can take different amount of pressure. Some bodies are very delicate, while they may not look that way, they can take only a little pressure, while a delicate looking body may ask for more pressure. Therefore it is important to ascertain the amount of pressure your client can take in severe pain condition

pressure should not be applied, just gentle rubbing or moderate pressure, even if your client asks for more.

4. **RHYTHM-** Rhythm comes out of experience, rhythmic massage, like rhythmic music, is soothing and energizing.

5. **SPEED -** Speed of your hands movement determines whether your massage is relaxing or energizing. As slow gentle movement help to relax the mind and the body however the fast movements are good to energize the body as it improves circulation.

BASIC MASSAGE MOVEMENTS- Aromatherapy massages do not require any hacking or cupping movements of Swedish massage. It is effective enough with gentle movements, however all movements are directed towards the heart. Basic massage movement include following steps-

1. **Effleurage** is a stroking movement performed with palms pushing the tissues with pressure towards the heart. Hands should be relaxed and in contact with the soft tissues using firm but gentle pressure. Once contact is made it must be maintained keeping continuous motion, placing one hand on the body before removing the other thus ending each sequence. Effleurage improves circulation, helps to spread the Essential Oils and enables the client get accustomed to the masseur.

2. *Petrisage-* forms the main and longest part of massage in aromatherapy. It includes the following movements:

   a. *Kneading-* this is a circular movement done with palms surface or thumbs; depending upon the area the pressure is determined. This movement helps to break down muscle tension as well as fatty deposits.

   b. *Picking up-* here the tissues is 'picked-up' from the bones i.e. the muscles are lifted, squeezed and relaxed without losing contact with the body. The tissues are lifted and moved alternatively, backward and forward in a smooth rolling movement, parallel to the bones. This movement is especially beneficial to reduce fatty tissues.

   c. *Wringing-* is similar to picking up but a much stronger movement. The flesh is lifted and wrung between both the hands. This is performed mostly on large muscle eg. thighs and buttocks.

3. *Friction -* helps to breakdown 'knotted-muscles. It also soothes nerve endings besides aiding distribution of fluid around joints eg. ankles. The movement involves the thumb working in circles with pressure on upward motion only.

FRICTION is combined or followed with Lymphatic Drainage- Friction helps moving the flow of lymph and blood, which should be drained to the nearest lymphatic nodes.

What is MLD?

Manual Lymphatic Drainage (MLD) is an advanced therapy in which the practitioner uses a range of specialized and gentle rhythmic pumping techniques to move the skin in the direction of the lymph flow. This stimulates the lymphatic vessels which carry substances vital to the defense of the body and removes waste products. The first visit will include a consultation during which the therapist will recommend the number and frequency of future sessions. Each session will last approximately one hour. It is appropriate that the therapist works in conjunction with your medical practitioner, in case of chronic or acute health conditions.

Benefits of MLD?

MLD is both preventative and remedial and can enhance your well being. Furthermore, MLD:

- is deeply relaxing
- promotes the healing of fractures, torn ligaments, sprains and lessens pain.
- can improve many chronic conditions: sinusitus, rheumatoid arthritis, scleroderma, acne and other skin conditions.
- may strengthen the immune system.
- relieves fluid congestion: swollen ankles, tired puffy eyes and swollen legs due to pregnancy.
- is an effective component of the treatment and control of lymphoedema and assists in conditions arising from venous insufficiency.
- promotes healing of wounds and burns and improves the appearance of old scars.
- minimizes or reduces stretch marks.

Aromatic oils can also be rubbed into particular areas of the body to help combat specific complaints: tense, aching shoulders should be kneaded using -a soothing massage oil to relax the muscles; stomach ache or period pain can be eased with gentle antispasmodic oil applied to the abdomen in a clockwise direction.

Massage can also be very intimate and sensual experience, between lovers, it can bring a new depth to a relationship, as well as enhance sexual enjoyment. Some essential oils like Jasmine, Ylang Ylang, Rose etc are renowned for their aphrodisiac effect!

For the purpose of massage, essential oils are mixed with a base oil or vegetable oil, such as sweet almond, olive or grape seed oil, before being applied to the body. The dilution should be in the region of 1-3 per cent depending upon the type of oil used and the specific purpose. In general, complaints of a physical nature, such as aching muscles or rheumatism, require a stronger concentration than disorders related to the emotions, like depression or insomnia.

You can use the blends below to nourish the body and mind. The stimulating blend can help to improve poor circulation and will revive you if you are tired or run down. Keep the soothing blend for evening use, since it will relax and prepare for sleep.

Soothing Blend	Stimulating Blend
2 drops of Geranium	3 drops of Lemon
3 drops of Lavender	2 drops of Rosemary
2 drops of Sandalwood	2 drops of Juniper Berry
1/2 fl oz (15 ml 2 1/2 tsp)	1/2 fl oz (15 ml 2 1/2 tsp)
of suitable carrier oil	of suitable carrier oil

Choose whichever blend appeals to you. Mix the essential oils with carrier oil and store in a clearly labeled screw top bottle.

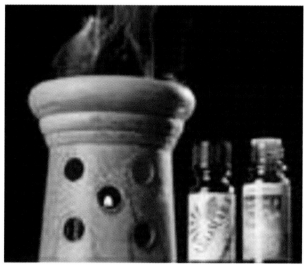

Vaporization:

Aromatherapy vaporizers are a quick and easy way to disinfect and make your environment smell beautiful. In a vaporizer oils are heated gently to evaporate from liquid to gaseous state filling the room with wonderful aromas. In past essential oils had been vaporized to prevent epidemics and spread of infectious diseases.

Vaporized oils can be used for a variety of reasons viz creating a relaxed atmosphere at home or uplift and stimulate minds in the office, disinfect the sick room etc. A penetrating oil like sweet basil, for example, can scent a room and dispel unwanted odours; while antiseptic oil such as eucalyptus can rid of room germs and combined with peppermint, will help with respiratory complaints; insect repellant aromas like citronella and lemongrass can be used to repel mosquitoes and other insects.

There are many ways to vaporize the oils. You can use an oil burner or an electric diffuser or simply add a few drops of oil to a bowl of hot water placed on a radiator. Avoid applying essential oils directly on to light bulb, as this may cause the bulb to explode. If you wish to keep insects at bay, applying oils to hanging ribbons or to clothing like curtain drapes etc, can be very effective. A few drops of an expectorant and decongestant essential oil such as Eucalyptus and Myrtle put on the pillow at night combat coughs and colds. Same way a combination of Mandarin and Marjoram will prevent snoring and combination of Clary sage with Marjoram will promote peaceful sleep. These are all ways of ensuring that the vaporized oils are used effectively.

Some useful oils for vaporization are as under-

RELAXING	UPLIFTING	SEDATIVE	SENSUAL
Lavender	Lemon	Clary sage	Jasmine
Sandalwood	Basil	Marjoram	Ylang Ylang
Vertivert	Neroli	Lavender	Patchouli
Geranium	Rosemary	Valerian	Cedar wood
Mandarin	Lemongrass	Patchoul	Clove

Steam Inhalation

An easy way to reap the benefits of essential oils is to inhale thems through steam vapors, the faster the oils evaporate, faster you breath them in and faster you get decongested, besides your skin also gets cleansed.

This method is especially suited to decongest sinus, throat and chest. Add about 5-10 drops of an essential oil, such as Eucalyptus, Rosemary or Peppermint or a combination of all, to a bowl of steaming water, cover the head with a towel and breathe deeply for 3-10 min keeping the eyes closed. Soaking in a steaming hot bath containing expectorant oils, which are non-irritating to the skin, such as the Pine needle or Marjoram, can also help clear congestion.

Do it in three simple steps:

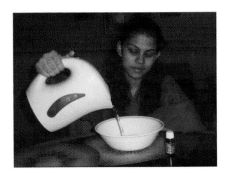 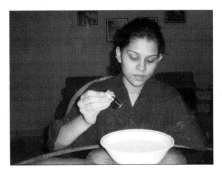 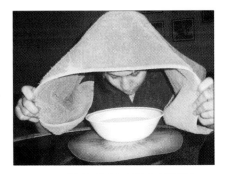

1.FILL A BOWL with STEAMING HOT WATER.   2.ADD 5-10 DROPS OF CHOSEN ESSENTIAL OILS.   3.INHALE THE STEAM USING A TOWEL TO SEAL IN THE VAPORS.

Steam inhalation also acts as a kind of facial "sauna". The use of oils such as Tea tree, Juniper berry, Geranium and Lavender can help unblock the pores and clear the complexion of spots and blackheads.

Steam inhalations are not recommended for asthma sufferers.

Compress

Compresses are simple and useful way of treating a wide range of body conditions with aromatherapy essential oils. From cuts, bruises and grazes to sprains, strains, inflammation, fever etc. essential oils used in compresses can help in wide range of problems and help in recovery process.

Compresses are simply a cloth or hand towel soaked in hot or ice cold water, to which essential oils are added. Hot and cold compresses are used to treat different conditions and it's important to know when to use which type of compress.

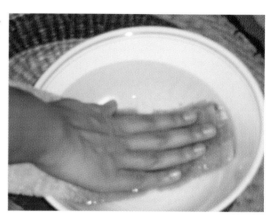

HOT COMPRESS

Hot compresses increase circulation to the affected area and help to relieve muscular aches and pains, arthritis and rheumatic pain, lower back pain, menstrual pain, frozen shoulder, muscle cramps, cystitis, abscesses etc. You can crush a piece of Ginger while heating the water, it increases heat and circulation.

Useful oils for compress are- *Eucalyptus, Ginger, Black pepper, Clove, Chamomile, Lavender, Wintergreen, Myrtle* etc.

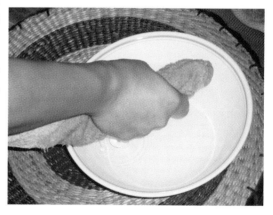

COLD COMPRESS

Cold compresses especially those incorporating ice help reduce swelling; they can be applied to relieve conditions like bumps, bruises, inflammation, boils, headaches, fever etc. Useful oils for cold compress are *Lavender, Rosemary, Eucalyptus, Peppermint, Basil* etc

You can also use hot and cold compresses alternating between the two for sprains, arthritis, boils etc.

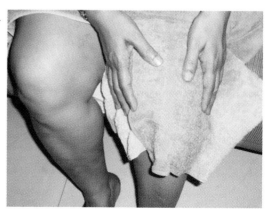

Foot Bath

Nothing is lovelier than an aromatic foot soak. Just a 10 minutes foot soak in warm water can help tired feet, swollen feet with edema or sweaty feet. You can simply use either your bath tub or any flat vessel to soak your feet in. For tired feet add 8 to 10 drops of Lavender, Rosemary and Basil. For swollen feet add 8 to 10 drops of Juniper berry, Cypress and Black pepper. For sweaty feet use Pine needles, Cypress and Eucalyptus.

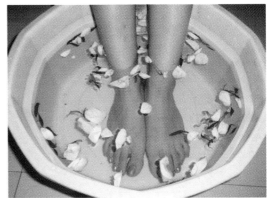

After foot bath dry your feet with a towel and apply few drops of either neat Lavender for tired and aching feet or use little Jojoba oil on dry feet.

Sitz Bath

Sitz baths are very useful for urinary, genital and anal complaints like cystitis, pruritis, thrush, haemarroids, piles, fistula.

Cystitis, which is an infection of the bladder, is characterized by a painful burning sensation while passing urine. Pruritis, or itching, is an irritating condition which often accompanies a mild vaginal infection. Best help for the condition is sitz bath with bactericidal oils, two to three times daily. They are easy to make simply add chosen essential oils to a tub of warm water, in which you can sit in. Alternatively you can use bath tub for the same purpose.

To help combat cystitis and pruritis. Add 5-10 drops of either Lavender, Juniper, Sandalwood, Tea tree, Cypress or Bergamot to sitz bath water, or add 2-3 drops to a bidet for local washing.

Douche

Douche is a vaginal enema in which we add essential oils. This method can be very helpful in the treatment of vaginal conditions, such as leucorrhea, candida, thrush or any other vaginal infection.

Here in you use plastic douche or an enema pot, Add 3-5 drops of any three of the following essential oils viz- *Tea tree, Sandalwood, Palmarosa, Cypress, Lavender, Juniper, Geranium* to warm water and stir well before inserting.

Gargle

For the treatment of mouth ulcers, sore throats, bad breath or other mouth or gum infections, simply add about 3 drops of an essential oil such as *Tea Tree, Cypress, Clove, Bergamot and Fennel* to glass of warm boiled water, mix well and gargle.

Neat Application;

Pure essential oils are strong chemicals and should not be applied neat to the skin. Some oils can cause irritation, a burning or tingling sensation when they are applied in an undiluted form; however there are exceptions to this rule. Lavender, for example, can be applied directly to burns, insect bites, cuts, cramps, tired or pulled muscles. Tea tree oil can be used directly on warts and nail bed infections. Some oils can be used as perfumes (like Sandalwood, Jasmine, Rose and Agarwood oil). Otherwise, most oils should never be applied undiluted, unless specifically directed. In case of emergency like a cut or wound, any oil can be used neat to have antiseptic effect.

Perfumes

In India and other parts of the worlds attars or traditional perfumes were being made with natural essential oils. Many essential oils are ideal as perfumes - either on their own or combined with others, such as Rose, Jasmine, Neroli and Sandalwood are very popular scents. Ylang Ylang, Patchauli and Geranium are renowned as well-balanced fragrances, they can be dabbed on the wrist or behind the ears (on the pulse points), either neat or diluted in 5 per cent of jojoba (for example 10 drops to 1 tsp of oil). Before using, a new oil, as a perfume, always do a patch test. Aromatic oils can also be used to scent hair, linen, clothes, paper, pot pourries or other items.

Pure essential oils have a totally different quality to synthetic perfumes because they are derived from natural sources. Artificially made perfumes do not have the subtle balance of constituents and the therapeutic qualities of real essential oils, besides causing allergic reaction in sensitive people.

Skin Care

Aromatherapy essential oils are ideally suited for skin care, since they are readily absorbed and have the ability to penetrate through to the underlying layers of the skin.

> Essential oils stimulate cellular regeneration, improve circulation and help to eliminate toxins at the fundamental level. Therefore the skin that has been treated with aromatic oils, thus become more dynamic and healthy. Therefore skin and beauty care are central to the practice of aromatherapy mostly practiced by beauty therapists or by oneself. Most of the aromatic recipes are simple and easy to make at home.

Facial Oils

These are blended in the same way as massage oils, except that the carrier oil, as well as the essential oil can be adapted to the type of skin being treated. Additional specialized base oils like Avocado, Jojoba, Wheatgerm, Hazelnut, Rosehip seed, Borage seed, Carrot macerated and Evening primrose may be used, in combination with the basic carrier oils such as sweet Almond, Grape seed, Sunflower, Sesame seed and Soya oil.

An easy recipe is 2 teaspoon of basic carrier oil with 1 teaspoon of specialized carrier oil suited to skin type and 6-8 drops of essential oil. (please refer to the Chapter on Face in next section for various facial formulations).

Facial Creams

An aromatic facial cream can be made by adding 8-10 drops of essential oil (according to skin type) to an unscented cream (100 gm jar) or by making up a basic cream for oneself, as under:

> 10 gm beeswax
> 40 gm almond oil
> 40 gm rose water/ distilled water
> 10 drops of chosen essential oil

Shred the beeswax and put it into Pyrex bowl together with the almond oil. Place the bowl in a double burner or a pan of water over gentle heat, and mix until the beeswax has melted. Warm the water in the same fashion, and add to the wax and the oil mixture bit by bit, beating all the time. On cooling of the cream mix add and stir in the essential oil and put in the fridge to set.

This cream can be used for the face, the hands or for massage to the body.

Gels-

Natural gels like Aloe vera or Witch hazel provide a useful non oily medium for the application of essential oils, as an alternative to oils and creams. A gel can be used to dilute any essential oil for irritating skin conditions, such as eczema or athlete's foot, particularly if the skin is broken, since they prevent the skin forming a crust. This method is also suitable for general skin care, especially if the skin tends to be greasy. Add 2-3 drops of essential oil to a teaspoonful of gel and mix well before applying to the skin.

Masks

Face masks have many benefits - they can nourish, rejuvenate, stimulate, cleanse, the skin, and generally improve its texture and wide range of natural ingredients and clay. There are many different fullers earth are the most versatile, in minerals. An essential oil and clay of acne and congested skin. Honey complexions, for helping to balance generally rejuvenating.

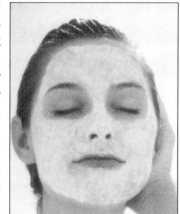

quality. Masks can be made from a including fruit pulp, yoghurt, honey types of clay, but green clay or as they are good antiseptic and rich mask is excellent for the treatment is also good for revitalizing dry combination skin, as well as being

An effective and easy recipe is given and Dry skin. Apply the mask once a improvement in skin texture.

hereunder for Normal-to-oily skin week to achieve a noticeable

Normal to Oily Skin
2 drops of Juniper
1 drop of Geranium
1 drop of Lavender
2 tsp of live, natural Yogurt

Dry Skin
1 drop of Sandalwood
1 drop of Lavender
1 drop of Roman chamomile
2 tsp of Honey

Blend the oils with the yoghurt or honey and spread the mixture lightly and evenly over the face. After a few minutes, when the mask no longer feels cool, rinse off and apply a moisturizer.

A good basic recipe is 50gms of green clay and 2 teaspoons of cornflower, mixed together and kept in jar. When you want to make a mask, mix 1 tablespoon of water and 3 drops of an essential oil suited to your skin type. Avoid clay masks for dry skin or after aromatherapy treatments unless you add little base oil to it, it will draw the moisture out of the skin.

Flower Waters-

These are easy to make and are beneficial for all types, of skin. Simply add up to 100 drops of essential oil to a 500 ml bottle of distilled or Rose water, leave it to stand for up to a month, and then filter using coffee filter paper. Lavender, Lemon, Rose and Neroli are the most traditional oils to make floral water but other oils such as Geranium or Sandalwood may also be used either individually or blended together.

A variety of essential oils can also be diluted in alcohol to make toilet waters, eau de-colognes or after shave lotions. For example, a traditional toilet water called Eau-de-Portugal, can be made by mixing, 20 drops of sweet Orange, 5 drops of Geranium in 1 tablespoon of vodka and 100 ml of spring water. Shake well and leave it to mature for a month at least and then filter.

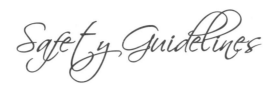

Safety Guidelines

Experiencing and exploring, the unique scents and individual properties of essential oils is both helpful and inspiring. In general, essential oils are safe to use, if used correctly. However, because of the high concentration and potency of the oils it is necessary to take some precautions into account, as you would with any other item. Some components of essential oils can also cause adverse effect on skin or mind.

Safety Data-

Always check the specific safety data and caution, before using a new oil.

Internal Use

Do not take essential oils internally. This rule is in accordance with the safety guidelines recommended by the International Federation of Aromatherapists. Essential oils don't mix with water, and in an undiluted form they may damage the delicate lining of the digestive tract. In addition, some essential oils are toxic, if taken internally. There is a misconception that things taken internally will work faster and better, that is not true as our digestive system is selective and does not absorb everything available while the skin is semi permeable and absorbs up to 40 % of essential oils when diluted in light base oils.

Neat Application

In general, essential oils should not be applied neat to the skin - always dilute them in a carrier oil, gel or cream first. There are exceptions to this rule, such as the use of neat Lavender for cuts, spots, burns, etc. also for emergency use. Certain non-irritant essential oils, can be made as perfumes. Always do a patch test first and keep well away from the eyes.

Skin Irritation

Oil which may irritate the skin or cause an allergic reaction are sweet Basil, Black Pepper, Cinnamon, Clove bud, Eucalyptus, Ginger, Lemon, Lemongrass, Peppermint, Pine needle and thyme. These oils should be used in half the usual recommended dilutions and no more than 3 drops added to the bath. If the irritation does occur, bathe the area with cold water.

Sensitive Skin

Some oils including Tea tree, may cause skin irritation in people with very sensitive skins. Since Tea tree is such a useful oil (which may sometimes be used neat), it is important for those with sensitive skins to dilute it first in non-oily cream or gel. Always do a patch test before using a new oil to check for individual sensitization.

Patch Test-

Before applying any new oil to the skin, even as a perfume, it is recommended to do a patch test. Simply put a few drops on the back of your wrist, cover with a plaster and leave for an hour or more. If irritation or redness occurs, bathe the area with cold water. For further use, reduce the concentration level by half or avoid the oil altogether,

Toxicity

Essential oils should be used in moderation and externally. Because of high toxicity levels certain oils like *Aniseed, Camphor, Clove bud, Hyssop, Nutmeg, Oregano, sweet Fennel and Spanish Sage* should be avoided or used in very small dosages.

Hazardous oils such as pennyroyal, mustard, sassafras, rue and mugwort should not be used at all.

Photo Sensitivity and Photo Toxicity

Some oils are photo toxic, which means they cause skin pigmentation if exposed to direct sunlight. Do not use the following oils on the skin, either neat or in dilution, if the area will be exposed to the sun or ultra-violet light (as on a sun bed): Bergamot (except bergapten-free oil), Angelica, Cumin, Lemon, Lime or Orange,

Babies and Children

Always dilute oils for babies and infants to at least half the recommended amount. For young children, avoid altogether the possible toxic and irritant oils listed above.

Babies 0-12 month: Use only 1 drop of Lavender, Geranium, Rose, Roman Chamomile, Neroli or Manderin essential oil, diluted in 1 teaspoon carrier oil for massage or bathing.

Infants 1-5 years: Use only 2-3 drops of the aforesaid "safe" oils i.e. those which are non-toxic and non-irritant, diluted in 1 teaspoon carrier oil for massage or bathing.

Children 6-12 years: Use as for adults but in half the stated concentration.

Teenagers: Use as directed for adults.

Pregnancy

During pregnancy, use essential oils in half the usual stated amount because of the sensitivity of the growing foetus. Oils which are potentially toxic or have hormonal or emmenagogic properties (that is, they stimulate the uterus muscles) are contraindicated.

The following oils should be avoided altogether: *Basil, Cinnamon leaf, Citronella, Clary sage, Clove, Hyssop, Juniper, Marjoram, Myrrh, Spanish Sage, Tarragon and Thyme.*

The following oils are best avoided during the first four months of pregnancy: *Atlas Cedarwood, Peppermint, Rosemary, Clary sage, Juniper berry and sweet Fennel.*

High Blood Pressure

Avoid the following oils, in case of high blood pressure or hyper-tension as they can raise the blood pressure level : *Hyssop, Rosemary, Cypress, Black Pepper, Sage (all types) and Thyme.*

Epilepsy

Most of the oils ,with high ketones and phenols contents, have strong aroma that can have strong effect on nervous system and may be neuro toxic for epileptics. The following oils should be used with care on epileptics, due to powerful effect on the nervous system: sweet Fennel, Hyssop, Peppermint, Thyme, Jasmine and Sage.

Alcohol

The oils of Clary sage and Marjoram, should not be used in any form within a few hours of drinking alcohol. It can cause nausea and exaggerated drunkenness.

Homeopathy

Homeopathic treatment is not compatible with the following oils due to their strength: Black Pepper, Camphor, Eucalyptus and Peppermint.

Storage

Store in dark bottles, way from light and heat, and well out oil reach of children.

Using aromatherapy with other therapies

All holistic therapies have been dubbed, as alternative therapies, in fact they are all complementary therapies and you can combine two or three systems of healing. The job of the healer is not to prove the supremacy of one therapy over the other, but to heal the client. In fact, use of essential oils has already been part of some of the ancient therapies like Ayurveda, essential oils can also be combined with modern medicine. Besides naturopathy, acupressure, Reiki, Pranic healing and other energy healing techniques can make use of the healing properties and high vibrations of the natural essential oils. I had personally been using essential oils for healing of chakras with chakras anointments.

CHAKRA HEALING WITH ESSENTIAL OILS

What human beings are to the animal world, a tree is to the plant kingdom. The five elements and three gunas, that we associate with various Chakras are also represented in plants. For that reason Ayurveda classifies certain plants and oils more Sattvic than others.

Five basic elements in Plants and use of their essences for chakra healing-

Earth- As earth element is associated with our root chakra, in plants it is associated with the roots. Similarly the oils from various plant roots are used to energize and balance the base root or Mooladhar chakra. Jatamansi (Indian spikenard) is a renowned essential oil used for Mooladhar as well as Crown chakra imbalances. Other useful oils are Angelica root, Valerian root, Costus root, Nagarmotha, Patchauli, Vertiver etc.

Water- Water element though associated with Swadhisthan or Sacral chakra is associated with the plant trunk, since trunk work as the water ways for the entire plant. Most useful, among the oils for Sacral chakra are Sandalwood, Cedar wood, Rose wood, Ginger (a modified stem) etc.

Fire- The fire element is represented in our Solar Plexus or Manipura chakra, it is associated with the brightly colored flowers and spices like Black pepper and Clove. Other useful oils are Rosemary, Marjoram, Chamomiles, Lavender, Thyme, Fennel, Cardamom, Rose, Geranium, Lotus, Clary Sage etc.

Air- The air element present in our heart chakra is represented in plants through its leaves. The most revered plant for heart chakra is Holy Basil, other useful plant oils are Eucalyptus, Peppermint, Lotus, Rose, Tea Tree, Lemongrass, Rosemary, Frankincense, Lavender, Thyme etc.

Ether- Described as space or akash tattva (element) is associated with our Vishudhha or Throat chakra.

In plant this element is associated with the fruits and the seeds. The useful oils are Lemon, Orange, Bergamot, Bayberry, Sandalwood, Lotus, Tea tree etc.

Our Third Eye chakra represents all the five basic elements (Panch mahabhoot), plant seeds also represent all the five elements. A seed is pure potentiality, of being a plant, the seed oils, according to their property can be used on all the chakras.

Essential oils can also be used for energy cleansing, aura cleansing and crystals cleansing. Some of my favourite oils for the purpose are Frankincense, Holy Basil (Tulsi), Sage, Rosemary, Myrrh etc. For chakra application essential oils should be diluted in a suitable base oil. Lotus seed or black til (Sesame seed) oil is considered as Sattvic base oils, to be used for chakra anointments. You can also combine oils for each chakras according to the therapeutic effect on the associated organs and glands or as per their colour vibrations. The selection and dosage should be as per the assessment of a qualified therapist having an understanding of chakra imbalances also. In case of doubts it is advised to use pre blended anointments, from a known source.

50 Easy ways of using Aromatherapy/Essential Oils

1. Essential oils in bath are the easiest and most versatile way. They work at physical as well as psychological level. At physical level they boost immune system while at psychological level they affect your mental / emotional state. Lavender and Geranium are most versatile all rounders which can be used to alone or in combination with other oils.

2. Keep hypertension at bay by using a combination of Lavender, Geranium, Sandalwood oil as a relaxing bath oil (5 drops in a bucket and 12-15 in bath tub), it will also boost immune level.

3. To lift mood and overcome depression use a combination of Lemon grass, Bergamot, Geranium and rosemary, you can use this combination in bath (5 drops in a bucket and 12-15 in bath tub) or vaporize.

4. Add a few drops of essential oils of Lemon grass, Rosemary, Lemon to water in a spray bottle and use as an air freshener. Add Rosemary, Frankincense, Holy Basil to cleanse the energy around.

5. To disinfect your home or a patients room, use few drops of Eucalyptus, Lemon, Cinnamon, Pine, Geranium and Tea Tree, either in a vaporizer or water sprayer.

6. Overindulged last night? Essential oils of Juniper, Cedarwood, Grapefruit, Lavender, Fennel, Rosemary, Peppermint and Lemon help soften the effects of a hangover. Make your own blend using 3-5 of these oils and use a total of 5-6 drops in bath.

7. Relieve muscle cramps with neat Lavender application. For tired aching muscles or arthritis aches, mix 1 part Eucalyptus, wintergreen, Lavender, Rosemary, Sage and Basil oil to 4 parts olive or other vegetable oil and use as a massage oil.

8. Ease headache/ migraine pain by rubbing a drop of Lavender with a touch of Peppermint oil onto your forehead and the back of your neck.

9. To blend your own massage oil, add 3-5 drops of your favorite essential oils to 1 oz. Jojoba or other skin-nourishing vegetable oil like Lavender, Geranium and Sandalwood. Don't make too much

10. First- aid for cuts, burns, bumps, insect bite even cramp or sprain use a combination of Lavender, Tea Tree and German chamomile.

11. For urinary infections use a combination of Tea tree, Sandalwood, Palmarosa and Juniper berry in sitz bath.

12. Smelly and sweaty feet can be remedied by either dropping a few drops of Pine Needle, cypress and Geranium essential oils directly into the shoes or by placing a cotton ball dabbed with a few drops of Lemon oil into the shoes or use the oils in a foot bath.

13. For Leucorrhea, candida & thrush use tea tree and lemon oil/ bergamot oil combination in sitz bath or douche.

14. For Quick relief from mouth ulcers dab 1 drop tea tree oil on two to three times in a day.

15. For bad breath use a combination of Bergamot, Geranium, Tea tree and Spearmint oil for gargle, twice daily.

16. For quick relief from laryngitis, pharingitis use a combination of Sandalwood, Tea tree, Lemon and Bergamot oil for gargle (with warm water) two to three times daily.

17. Apply true Lavender oil and Tea tree oil directly to cuts, scrapes, or scratches. 1 or 2 drops will promote healing.

18. Lavender, Clary sage and Marjoram promote sleep and relieve insomnia, use a few drops on your pillows or night suit collar.

19. Lavender helps reducing blood pressure and hypertension, it can also be a good first aid to a heart attack patient, rub on chest and soles of feet.

20. Dab your acne / pimples or any boil with Tea tree oil for quick result.

21. Place 1 drop of Peppermint oil in 1/2 glass of water, sip slowly to relieve hot flushes, it also aids digestion and relieve upset stomach.

22. For quick relief from asthma attack, inhale peppermint oil.

23. For any skin allergy use Lavender oil with a few drops of water.

24. Combination of Lavender, Marjoram and Clary sage in a vegetable oil massaged on lower abdomen relieve menstrual cramps.

25. 1 drop of Tea Tree or Oregano essential oils applied directly to a wart is an effective means of elimination. Apply the essential oil daily until the wart is gone.

26. For nail bed infections use a drop of Tea tree oil for a few days until it's gone.

27. Rosemary oil helps people suffering from low blood pressure, use in bath or massage.

28. Rosemary also promotes alertness and stimulates memory. Inhale occasionally during long car trips and while reading or studying.

29. To relieve anxiety, lie down on bed and use a few drops of lavender oil on your solar plexus, mothers can use it for the children.

30. For quick relief for sprained and stiff muscles - Apply Lavender oil directly.

31. Potpourri which has lost its scent can be revived by adding a few drops of essential oil add Patchouli and Sandalwood for longer lasting effect.

32. The bathroom is easily scented by placing oil-scented cotton balls in inconspicuous places or sprinkle oils directly onto silk or dried flower arrangements or wreaths.

33. Essential oils or blends make wonderful perfumes. Create your own personal essence using 25 drops of essential oils to 1 oz of perfume alcohol. Let it age two weeks before using.

34. Essential oils dropped on a radiator, scent ring, or light bulb will not only fill the room with a wonderful fragrance, it will also set a mood such as calming or uplifting.

35. When moving into a new home, first use a water spray containing a combination of Basil, Sage,

Rosemary & Frankincense essential oils they will cleanse the aura and change the odorous environment to your own. Do this for several days until it begins to feel like your space.

36. To bring fever down, sponge the body with cool water to which 1 drop each of Eucalyptus, Peppermint, and Lavender oils have been added.

37. Jojoba oil makes ideal hair nourisher for colored hair, without affecting the color. It can also be used on eye brows.

38. When washing out the fridge, freezer, or oven, add 1 drop of Lemon, Lime, Grapefruit, Bergamot, Mandarin, or Orange essential oil to the final rinse water.

39. To dispel mosquitoes and other picnic or Bar-B-Q pests, drop a few drops of Lemongrass or Citronella oil with Camphor in the melted wax of candle or place a few drops on the Bar-B-Q hot coals.

40. Infuse bookmarks and stationary with essential oils. It will save them from moth and silverfish. Place drops of oil on paper and put them in a plastic bag, seal it and leave overnight to infuse the aroma. Send only good news in perfumed letters.

41. Use 1 drop Roman Chamomile oil on a cloth wrapped ice cube to relieve teething pain in children.

42. To fragrance your kitchen cabinets and drawers, place a "food scent" or Lemon oil dabbed on a cotton ball in an inconspicuous corner. To repel cockroaches use Camphor and Eucalyptus combination.

43. Add 1 drop each of Lavender, Geranium and Sandalwood oil to your facial moisturizer to bring out a radiant glow in your skin.

44. Place 1 or 2 drops of Rosemary or Ylang Ylang, on your hair brush before brushing to promote growth and thickness.

45. To enjoy a scented candle, place a drop or two of essential oil into the hot melted wax as the candle burns.

46. To dispel household cooking odors, add a few drops of Clove or Cinnamon oil to a simmering pan. 1 drop of Lemon essential oil on a soft cloth will polish copper with gentle buffing.

47. To make a natural flea collar, saturate a short piece of cord or soft rope with Pennyroyal or Tea Tree oil, roll up in a handkerchief and tie loosely around the animal's neck.

48. Put a few drops of your favorite essential oil on a cotton ball and place it in your vacuum cleaner bag it will give pleasant odor to your room. Lemongrass, Eucalyptus, Rosemary and Geranium are nice.

49. A wonderful massage blend for babies is 1 drop Roman Chamomile, 1 drop Lavender, 1 drop Geranium diluted in 2 tablespoons Sweet Almond oil and 1 tablespoon of Grape Seed Oil.

50. For Scent-Sational smelling towels, sheets, clothes, etc. place a few drops of Lavender, Geranium or any other chosen essential oil onto a small piece of terry cloth and toss into the clothes dryer while drying. Add 5 drops essential oil to 1/4 cup fabric softener or water and place in the center cup of the wash.

Section III

Aromatic Body & Beauty Therapy

Concept of Health & Beauty
Understanding Our Skin
Essential oils & our lymphatic system
The Face
Head & Hair Care
The Breasts
The Back & Shoulders
Tummy, Waist & Abdomen
Thighs & Buttocks
Knees, Ankles & feet
Upper Arms, Elbow & Neck
Hand & Nail Care

Aromatic Beauty & Body Therapy

This section on 'Aromatic Beauty & Body Therapy' is designed to examine various aspects of Health and Beauty. The balancing, cleansing and regenerative qualities of essential oils bring about a harmony of mind and body besides a healthy glow on the skin.

According to the ancient law of the "microcosm and macrocosm" there is no real difference between the vast external universe and limited universe of the human body. A human being is the living microcosm of the universe and universe is the macrocosm of a human being.

As per Kundalini Tantra, the human body is composed of three layers (bodies), which function as the vehicle for the inner self. These are not bodies in physical sense, rather a kind of energy sheath or vibratory field, which embodies the underlying consciousness. The physical body originates in the sexual union of the parents, this body we normally experience and sustain with food. Our awareness within this body constitutes the waking state of consciousness. It is made up of sixteen components- five sensory organs, five organs of action, five elements and the mind. The energetic basis or pure form of the physical body is subtle or astral body, represented as our AURA. The subtle body is also composed of sixteen components. Within the subtle body exist, the seven major Chakras, known as psychic energy centers.

Chakras, the energy centers, are transfer points for our thoughts, emotions and affect the physical functioning of our endocrine glands and vital organs. Chakra activity is affected by mental and emotional state, when they are balanced we feel maximum vitality, health and body ecstatic. Daily stress can result in Chakra imbalances and physical, physiological and emotional disorders.

HOLISTIC HEALTH- Our health is not, just the absence of disease rather it's the balance of the mind, body and the spirit. According to Ayurveda the ancient Indian science of health and healing it's the balance of five elements- earth, water, fire, air and ether, three gunas- Tamas, Rajas and Sattva, and three Doshas- Kapha, Pitta, Vata.

There are two concepts of medicine which are complementary to each other, though head and tail of the same coin. Orthodox (allopathic) medicine or classical medicine looks on sickness as "accidental"- a combination of signals and symptoms due to an exterior damaging agent. However, a complementary therapist would see the symptoms in the light of whole being - as clues to causes of the disease and to treat this rather than symptoms. The cause may lie in any of the different aspects of patient's life style viz. - a real disease or imbalance.

Self discipline is the key to healthy lifestyle that guarantees long lasting vigor and vitality. By following the healthy regimen you can promote health and avoid disease. The holistic approach is to look for the underlying causes of the disease by analyzing person's lifestyle and to treat these rather than symptoms. Over 80 % of health problems can be taken care of at home until they become chronic. Therefore it's important to look into the different aspects of the patient's life style viz;

a. **Mental / Emotional Lifestyle**- Mental attitudes play a far greater part in day to day health than is realized. For those who find positive thinking difficult or cannot have faith strong enough to believe that things can be changed, essential oils are an alternative route. Since, essential oils affect our health from the same starting point as our thoughts - the pituitary and the pineal body, the seat of the mind and emotions.

Negative thoughts and emotions adversely affect body's energy level and immune system. Emotional blocks mostly affect our sacral, heart and throat chakras and may lead to diseases associated with this chakras. Mental stress and anxieties affect our solar plexes chakra mainly and may also affect root and throat chakras.

"Psycho-neuro-immunology" is a fairly new discipline, it is the study of thoughts and how they can influence the brain, and directly affect health of our cells in all parts of the body and one's whole outlook of life. As an extension much emphasis is placed now-a-days on the relationship between our health and emotional state. 'We are what we think'- happy positive thoughts exert a positive influence on both health and life in general, whereas negative emotions are self-inflicted wounds which effectively close down the immune system leaving the body vulnerable to a wide range of psycho somatic disorders.

b. **Nutritional Lifestyle**- Diet and nutrition is an important factor for a healthy life. Incorrect eating habits could again be a cause of poor health and the saying 'You are what you eat' is indeed true.

c. **Physical Lifestyle**- Physical regimen also is the key to good health. Light exercises like yoga, Tai Chi etc have soma psychic (body over mind) effect and ease depression, assist in bowl movement, promote sound sleep. Exercises tone muscles, strengthen bones, make the heart and lungs work better and increase our physical reserve and vitality. Some people achieve the amount of exercise required from their normal routine while those who lead sedentary life style are prone to illness.

d. **Social life style**- A person's social life style is also responsible for his/her well being. While acceptability in a peer group or social circle leads to good health, living in solitude or heavy smoking/drinking regularly in groups or solitude is harmful for health.

e. **Spiritual life style**- Spirituality is the science of the SELF, our spiritual practices help us to manage our stress much better. If you notice, that those who are truly spiritual, have a certain radiance about them, they are much more in control of their mind and emotions. Therefore assessment of spiritual lifestyle is an important part of health assessment and guidance.

A complementary therapist has to look into all these aspects of a patient life style. Every disease can be cured but not every patient. There are people who enjoy being ill they don't really want to be cured, they enjoy sympathy and attention given to them. This is mostly a result of long-standing imbalance or insecurity in them.

HOLISTIC BEAUTY- is the beauty of the whole individual (man/ woman) not just the outer f the skin. The real beauty merges with inner beauty (which we can call spirit or love or compassion) with outer beauty, which is our physical body. The most beautiful woman is the one blessed with an attractive physical appearance, but above and beyond this she radiates love, joy contentment and good health.

Understanding Our Skin

One of the greatest treasures that a woman or man can have is healthy radiant skin. A beautiful complexion and glorious body skin are a reflection of our inner health and personal life style practice. In fact inner health is the sum total of our life styles- physical, nutritional, mental/emotional, social and spiritual.

The skin is a living organ and the largest of the body's organs. The whole skin of an adult had an area of about 2 square metres (20 sq. ft.). In total it weighs about 3 Kg (61/2 lb). Just one square inch has 94 sebaceous glands, 60 hairs, 19,000 sensory nerve cells, 1250 pain receptors and 19 yards of blood vessels.

It is made up of two main layers: the epidermis which you see and the dermis. The epidermis makes up the top half-millimeters (1/50 in.) or so. Beneath this is the dermis, about 2 millimeters (2/25 in thick).

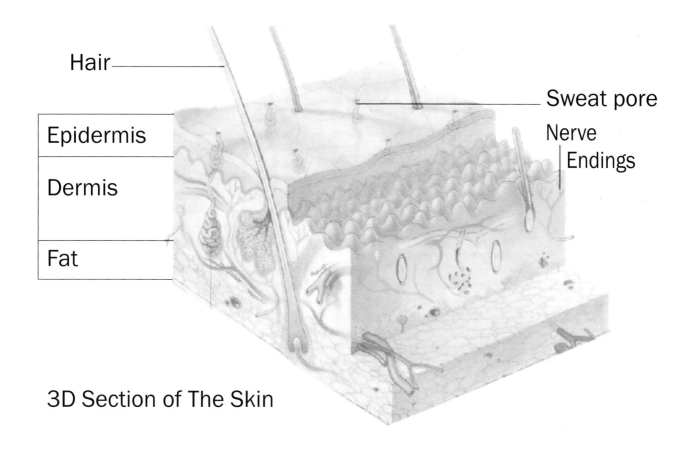

Hair

Sweat pore

Nerve
Endings

Epidermis

Dermis

Fat

3D Section of The Skin

Millions of dividing cells at the base of the epidermis push wave after wave of new cells towards the surface. Closer to the surface, they are squashed flat and, this flexible pavement of dead cells is waterproof. The outer layer protects by sealing in all the body's fluids and keeping out potentially harmful things. The inner layer supports, nourishes and supplies it with that most essential commodity – moisture. In structure the two layers are different, the epidermis consists of several rows of living cells covered by compact sheets of dead cells (sometime referred to as keratin layer). It is constantly growing and about every twenty days new cells are born at its base. They quickly die and dead cells are then pushed to the surface by the arrival of the new ones underneath and are continuously shed. Every new top layer is another chance to have a beautiful skin. Even if you remove a portion of the outer layer it will grow back as good as new. The dermis gives the skin its strength and ability to stretch. It is here that vital nerves, glands, hair follicles and blood vessels are to be found. Skin contains millions of sensitive nerve endings which tell the brain about touch, temperature, pressure and pain. Sebaceous glands produce oil, called sebum which keeps the skin supple and waterproof. The different structures in the skin work together, to help control the body's temperature and receive touch sensations.

The living reproductive cells are nourished through the blood vessels, but the dead cells have only one requirement- water. It will plump, soften or smooth. The amount of water the outer layer holds determines the skin's texture and to some extent its contour. It receives a steady supply of water from the dermis, but this is limited and frequently not enough. The epidermis also holds the skin's pigment, the darker the skin, more the pigmentation, sebaceous and sweat glands, are situated below but communicating to the outer layer through ducts that end on the surface. Oil glands greatly influence the skin condition and skin type.

Our skin serves the body in many ways viz.

- Sensory perception.
- Protecting underlying tissues from injury and dehydration.
- Assisting in processes of temperature maintenance and toxic waste elimination.
- Serving as the origination point for the manufacture of Vitamin D.
- Giving structure to all organs and systems within the body.

Skin is the integral part of our being and plays a vital role within your body's supportive and functional capacities. It is essential that we learn to take care of it and nourish it so that it will remain healthy regardless of the climate we live in or our chronological age. Truly beautiful skin is always the result of healthy, stress free lifestyle and regular nourishing and cleansing. Nature has blessed us with a variety of products like essential and base oils used in aromatherapy and wholesome ingredients, many of which are available in our kitchen cupboard or fridge or available easily with a natural products supplier. You can use these products to create a variety of products to both cleanse and nourish your skin, hair, nails and more.

There are three skin types- OILY, DRY and balanced viz. NORMAL, many skins are a combination of oily and dry. What your skin needs in the way of treatment and preparations depends upon its type. Colour of the skin influences the texture and all skin types can have a sensitive or blemished condition.

OILY SKIN- *is mainly due to overactive sebaceous glands, affects mostly the dark skin, but the lighter skin are also affected. Excess oil causes skin to shine constantly, makes it coarse with enlarged pores. It is prone to acne, often gets black / white heads and occasional break outs. The only consolation is that it stays younger looking, longer, has few wrinkles and usually improves with age. Trying to remove all oils from the skin only encourages greater gland activity, so it's important to remove only the excess oil from surface, as too enthusiastic a treatment with harsh soap or cleansing lotion will often dehydrate the epidermis, leaving skin in a flaky condition.*

DRY SKIN- *Three different things cause dry skin, dehydration, insufficient amount of oil secretion and aging. Dry skin is generally of a fine texture, but looks and feels tight and drawn. It chaps, flakes and peels easily and even at an early age may show wrinkles and lines, particularly around the eyes and mouth. Best way to deal with dry skin is to try and avoid further dehydration by sealing the moisture or re-hydration. The lack of natural oils must be compensated by rich external lubrication.*

NORMAL or BALANCED SKIN- *This type of skin exists when oil, moisture and acidity are harmonious. It is ideal but rare. This type of skin is fine textured with no visible pores, smooth to touch, neither it's wet nor greasy. It has a tendency to become more dry, with time (aging) so it needs care to maintain status quo.*

COMBINATION SKIN- *This is really skin in transition between dry and oily state. It gives off too much oil in the T - area of forehead. Nose and chin, the rest is dry particularly around eyes and on cheeks. The dry and oily areas have to be treated separately.*

CONDITIONS :

Sensitive – Usually dry skin plus fine textured, often with a transparent look, the upper layer being particularly thin and sensitive and likely to develop broken capillaries as in case of rosacea. Reacts quickly, to both external and internal influences- sun, wind, emotions, food, drink. Needs usual dry skin care plus extra protective, gentle lubrication. Watch for any allergies.

Blemished- Usually oily skin plus troubled with pimples. Sometimes to the intensity of acne, needs usual oily skin care plus attention from medicated preparations that dry and heal- and professional advice. Sometimes skin gets blemished develops pigmentation due to hormonal imbalances, as in case of menopausal women.

COLOUR:

The colour of the skin depends on the degree of pigmentation. Light skin tones are graded from pale to pink, beige to rosy, dark skin tones go from olive to caramel, brown to black. There is no basic difference in structure or quality. Dark skin generally has more sweat and sebaceous glands hence more oily. The sun is the great enemy of light skins which usually have dry tendencies, so lines are created faster. The evenly distributed pigment in dark skins acts like a sun filter and it's more oily surface acts as a shield, keeping moisture in. Dark skins, even the black skin can tan and burn but less drastically than light skin. Dermatologists say, that black skin are less likely to develop acne or skin cancer.

Our skin is constantly renewing itself and it takes about 30 days for a newly formed skin cell to move step by step through the layers of epidermis until it becomes cornified and stratifed (hard & flat) and eventually is rubbed off the surface. Vitamin A controls the rate of cornification and anyone suffering from Vitamin A deficiency will have hard, horny skin. When we apply massage oils to the top layer, the epidermis, the tiny molecules of essential oil penetrate to the dermis (or corium) where the elasticity of the skin is governed. It is in this layer that fibres of collagen, elastic fibres and fibres of connective tissues are intermingled and it is the alignment of these fibres that gives the skin its elasticity. Also in this layer are the hair roots, gland, blood vessels and lymph vessels. A complex structure indeed, which gives us the word "COMPLEXION".

According to doctors Robert and Elizabeth McCarter, contributing authors of "The Life Science Health System" - A healthy skin sings of a well nourished body, of systemic equilibrium, of balance, of homeostasis, of sound living practices, of good inheritance, of vitality, of a clean, free flowing unobstructed blood stream, and of organs functioning silently and efficiently in a body as peace.

The skin is one of the first organs of the body to be affected by poor diet, vitamin and mineral deficiencies and improper elimination. In short, it's the mirror of your health. Moist, clear radiant skin is generally a sign of good health, while skin that is dry and flaky, or oily and pimply can be indicative of internal problems, especially where nutrition is concerned.

Remember; Nature's promise.......

TAKE CARE OF YOUR SKIN

And

YOUR SKIN WILL REWARD YOU

WITH HEALTH AND BEAUTY

FOR THE REST OF YOUR LIFE!

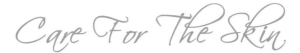

Care For The Skin

To keep your skin deep-down clean, no matter whether it's oily, combination, normal or dry, all that is necessary is that you observe these five basic practices, cleansing, toning, moisturizing , high water intake and dry brushing.

1. **CLEANSING-** A very important step, to be followed twice a day, using a wash cloth or facial sponge, apply the appropriate facial cleanser for your skin type, to your face and throat, to be massaged gently using upward, circular strokes. This step should be about a minute then rinse your face with clean warm water to remove all traces of the cleanser and pat dry. Aromatic cleansers are better as they do not disturb skin's pH. Never use a harsh or strong scrub on your facial skin- always be gentle.

2. **TONING-** A toner is designed to remove any traces of cleanser that have been left behind and restore the pH balance of the skin. Herbal liquids or aromatic waters make very gentle toners, just soak a cotton ball with it and apply in gentle , upward strokes. No need to pat dry- go on to moisturize.

3. **MOISTURIZING-** It's important even for oily skin. A moisturizer is designed to prevent dehydration (loss of water) of the skin. Even an oily skin can suffer from lack of water. A good moisturizer serves as a barrier between your skin and the environment. It will help to keep the skin younger looking for longer time. Simply apply the appropriate moisturizer after toner or otherwise, using upward, circular strokes until the moisturizer disappears.

4. **WATER INTAKE-** Sufficient water intake is essential to maintaining soft, moist, glowing skin. It can be in any form either plain water, fruit juices or raw fruits and vegetables.

5. **DRY BRUSHING-** A MUST for smooth, clear skin. Over the course of a day, our skin eliminates more than a pound of waste through thousands of tiny sweat glands. In fact, about one third of all the body's impurities are excreted this way. But if our pores are clogged by tight-fitting clothes, aluminium contained synthetic anti perspirants / deos, mineral based moisturizers, there is no way for these toxic byproducts, to escape, and the toxins have to seek another route to escape from body, causing skin to look pale, pasty, pimply or diseased. So the solution is DRY BRUSHING.

As the name suggests dry brushing is performed on dry skin- not oiled, not damp but dry before you shower. Use a natural fiber brush for gentle brushing not harsh on entire body except face and breasts. Begin brushing your hands, in between the fingers, then arms, underarms, neck, chest, stomach, back, then on to each leg beginning with the feet. You'll feel wonderfully invigorated when finished and your skin will glow. Use a light aromatherapy moisturizer or

Essential Oils & Our Lymphatic System

The body's lymphatic system is a vitally important component in the maintenance of good health. It is a network of vessels which reach almost every part of the body. The system collects plasma & white cells that have leaked out of the blood capillaries into the spaces between the body cells. The plasma and the white cells (together called the lymph) are squeezed into the lymphatic vessels as muscles contract. Lymph returns to the blood via a vein near the heart.

Lymph nodes are converging points of various lymphatic vessels, these nodes are swelling found in the groin, armpit, neck and elsewhere. White cells in these nodes fight infection by destroying bacteria. The nodes may become enlarged if the body is actively fighting an infection.

Lymph permeates all the body tissues, removing toxins and carrying infection fighting lymphocytes, to wherever they are needed. Before toxins are excreted from the body, they must firstly pass through the lymph nodes where they are broken down and then fed into the blood stream, from where they pass to the organs of elimination, and to make their way out of the body. When essential oils enter the body through the skin, either by massage, masks, bathing or any other method, they mix with lymph and carried along on the same journey as the toxins. During this journey, the antiseptic, anti-viral, anti-biotic or anti-fungal properties of essential oils are able to kill

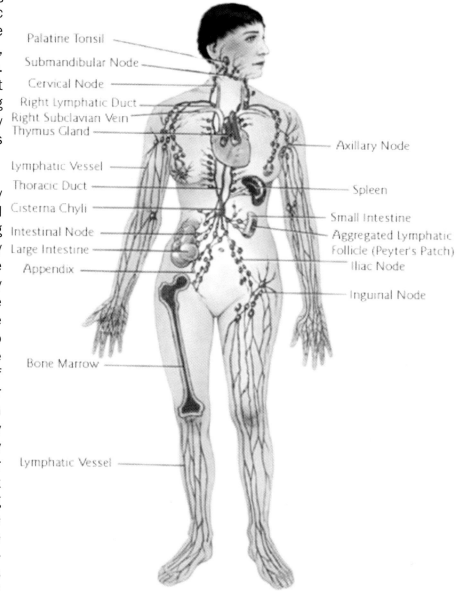

Palatine Tonsil
Submandibular Node
Cervical Node
Right Lymphatic Duct
Right Subclavian Vein
Thymus Gland
Lymphatic Vessel
Thoracic Duct
Cisterna Chyli
Intestinal Node
Large Intestine
Appendix
Bone Marrow
Lymphatic Vessel

Axillary Node
Spleen
Small Intestine
Aggregated Lymphatic Follicle (Peyter's Patch)
Iliac Node
Inguinal Node

off harmful organisms even before they reach the lymph nodes. Because there is less infective material passing into the lymph nodes, they rarely become inflamed and are better equipped to carry out their second function, which is to produce lymphocytes.

The lymph also carries away fluids and fats from body tissues and organs - a function which prevents us from becoming obese and water logged. Because essential oils perform an important role in keeping infection under control, the lymphatic system is able to carry off fats and fluids more easily, which means that our body's shape, as well as our health improves.

The lymphatic system is a part of the circulatory system and as such, is influenced by the heart. All the body systems are all inter connected, and according to the laws of acupuncture it is the lungs that govern the waterways of the body. The waterways refer to the lymphatic system, which means that as long as we are breathing, lymph is circulating around our body. It also means that any form of exercise that increases the action of the lungs is beneficial to the lymphatic system. Physical movement of the skin, such as the skin brushing or massage, is also very beneficial to the free flow of lymph.

There are many health problems that may result from congested and stagnant lymphatic system. Here is partial list of conditions that may improve with increased lymph flow:

Arthritis	Ovarian & Uterine Cysts	Headaches
Backaches	Fibrocystic Breasts	Migraines
Asthma	Painful & enlarged breasts	IBS (Irritable Bowel Syndrome)
Breast Cancer	Congested Lungs	Kidney problems
Cellulite	Congestive Heart Failure	Lymphoma
Chronic Fatigue	Crows Feet	Lymphoedema
Prostate Enlargement	Wrinkles	Neck & shoulder stiffness
Psoriasis	Dandruff	PMS
Rheumatism	Dizziness – Vertigo	Polyps
Ringing in Ears	Earaches	Skin disorders
Sagging chin	Edema	Eye diseases & poor vision
Sinus problems	Enlargement of Heart	Frequent Colds & Flu
Sluggishness	Excessive tiredness	Toxin Accumulation Heart
Obesity		Excessive tiredness

MANUAL LYMPHATIC DRAINAGE-

 MLD involves light, rhythmical massage that aids the body in collecting and moving lymphatic fluid, which plays a key role in delivering nutrients, antibodies and other immune constituents to the tissue cells of the body and removing debris such as toxins, cell waste and dead particles which are then cleansed by clusters of lymph nodes. MLD also works on the nervous system, lowering blood pressure, reducing stress and improving sleep patterns.

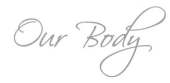

Our Body

The human body is a fascinating and remarkable machine. Its design is far more complex than the most advanced computer. Deep inside the body are billions of cells carrying out thousands of different functions, without our conscious knowledge, the body regulates its temperature and water content, the rate of the heart beat and numerous other processes. The coordinating centre for all these activities is the brain. It receives records and stores a greater variety of data than any computer ever could.

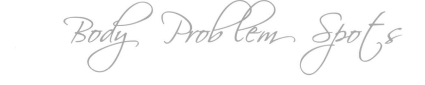

Body Problem Spots

Common external problems and problem areas in different body parts can be classified as under –

I. **THE FACE-** Dry and dehydrated skin, greasy skin, open pores, maturing skin, lifeless skin; double-chin; pimples and pimple marks, pigmentation & blemishes, tired and irritated eyes, dark circles, crow's feet, thin eyelashes, dry and chapped lips.

II. **HAIR & HEAD-** Dry lack luster hair, brittle hair, dandruff, excess grease; hair loss, tension in head, stressed-out feeling.

III. **BACK & SHOULDERS-** Congested, blemished skin, greasy skin, dull looking skin, tension in neck and shoulders.

IV. **BREASTS-** Sagging Breasts, Fibrocystic breast condition (lumps in breast), breasts too large or too small, stretch-marks, blemishes.

V. **UPPER ARMS, NECK & ELBOWS-** Flabby upper arms, cellulite, excess fat, wrinkled elbows, rough elbows, dry skin,

VI. **TUMMY & WAIST-** Excess fat, Wrinkles, Stored tension in solar plexus.

VII. **THIGHS & BUTTOCKS-** Cellulite, Obesity, Stretch marks, Buttocks droop, dull and lifeless skin.

VIII. **KNEES, ANKLES & FEE**T- Fat knees, puffy knees, wrinkly knees, puffy ankles, hidden ankles, tired feet.

IX. **HANDS & NAILS-** Dry skin dehydrated skin, fat or puffy hands, brittle nails, ridged nails.

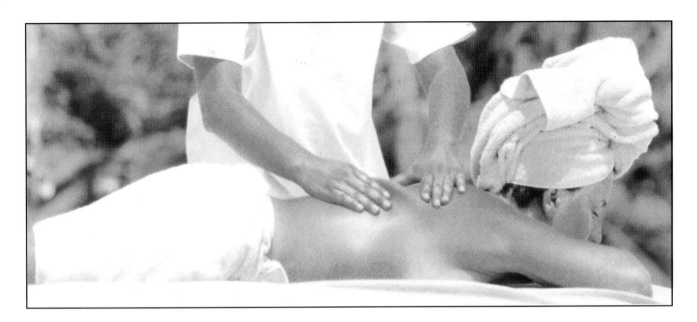

Each person is having different problem spots to be worked upon. So, the first objective is to identify and categorize the problem spots. Take into account the age, bone structure, genetics (hereditary factor) and life style of the person. If the person is large or big boned, don't imagine that massage with essential oils will make him/her look petite.

Categorize these problem spots into Major (Primary), Moderate (secondary) and Minor (tertiary) - and make an evaluation chart as under so as to evaluate the progress from time to time. After listing these conditions, list below them what is required to reverse the conditions for example – if we analyze a DRY, Mature Skin with pigmentation, we'll list them as under.

	Primary Condition	Secondary Condition	Tertiary Condition
Conditions -	Dry SKIN	Mature / aging	Pigmentation
Solutions -	Moisturize	Rejuvenate	Regulate Hormones

Now list all essential oils which are suitable for each category and choose the best five available with you for doing a blend.

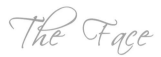

The Face

The Problems- *Dry and dehydrated skin, greasy skin, open pores, maturing skin, lifeless skin; double-chin; pimples and pimple marks & blemishes, tired and irritated eyes, dark circles, crow's feet, thin eyelashes, dry and chapped lips.*

The Causes- *Lack of natural oils or excess secretion of sebum, insufficient water, smoking and lack of nourishment (inside out); polluted environment; sun, stress and hormonal imbalance.*

The Solutions- Massage oils to feed and nourish the skin, re-hydration of the skin with aromatic waters and rebalancing oils, cleansing and rejuvenating (face lift) massage, friction massage, facial masks and facial steaming and cleansing regime for skin, decongesting oils, soothing aromatic compresses, toning the eye area, nourishing oils for lashes & brows, softening and protecting lip balms.

Care for the Face

Although there is saying that "Don't judge a book by its cover", in reality we are often judged by the look of our face, whether we are beautiful, attractive or plain, it can be seen on our faces. The mind is mirrored in the face and when 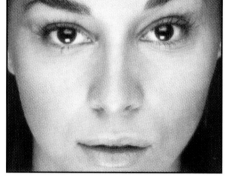 mentally stressed our face loses its attractiveness. When we feel happy & contented, a certain glow comes from within, which not only makes us feel good but is visible to others also.

Essential oils are ideally suited to skin care, for they are readily absorbed and have the ability to penetrate through to the underlying layers of the skin which are alive and active, unlike the outer dead layer of the cells that are constantly being shed. Essential oils stimulate cellular regeneration, improve the circulation and help to eliminate toxins at fundamental level. Skin that has been treated with essential oils thus becomes more dynamic and healthy. In addition, since the oils are able to travel in the blood stream and lymphatic system, skin treatments using essential oils are vitalizing to the body as a whole.

For Skin Care, not only the choice of correct essential oils is important, base oils are equally important. While essential oils provide the therapeutic benefits to the skin the vegetable oils provide the nourishment. As most of the vegetable oils are containing essential fatty acids (also called vitamin F) and other essential vitamins and minerals. The list of important essential / career oils for skin & hair care is given as under-

Important Essential Oils

1. LAVENDER
2. GERANIUM
3. FRANKINCENSE
4. TEA TREE
5. SANDALWOOD
6. CLARY SAGE
7. JUNIPER BERRY
8. ROSEMARY
9. GERMAN & Roman CHAMOLMILE
10. PALMAROSA
11. VERTIVER
12. ROSE
13. NEROLI
14. PETITGRAIN
15. CYPRESS

Important Base Oils

1. ALMOND-
2. OLIVE
3. WHEATGERM
4. JOJOBA
5. GRAPE SEED
6. EVENING PRIMROSE
7. AVACADO
8. HAZEL NUT
9. Macerated Carrot Oil
10. Calendula
11. FM's Career oil for Oily Skin
12. FM's Career Oil for Dry Skin

Mystery of PH

The natural acid/ alkaline balance of healthy skin has a pH (Potential Hydrogen) value of less than 7 it is acidic; when it is more than 7 it is alkaline. Most synthetic detergents and soaps are alkaline and can upset the natural acid mantle which protects against germs, dirt and invasive bacteria. It is therefore important that you do not strip the skin of this protective mantle and only use substances like essential oils which have neutral pH value (between 6.5-7).

Oily & Greasy skin-

Greasy skin is only a problem after the onset of puberty and before this turning point in our lives, the majority of us have smooth childhood skin. At birth we have approximately 100 sebaceous (oil producing) glands on every square centimeter of our skin with the exception of the soles of our feet, palms of our hands and the eardrum, but immediately after birth these glands are much more intense – up to 900 per square centimeter on the face, scalp, forehead and genital region.

Our sebaceous glands produce a thick, oily colorless secretion produced in cells or lobes, which break down and empty their contents in ducts which in turn empty into follicles. The life span of each one of these lobes is only about a week, but is an ongoing process, which lubricates the skin continually.

The composition of sebum is a complex, it is a mix of hundreds of fatty acids- a significant proportion of them being the well known fatty acids- palmitic, mysristic, stearic, oleic and linoleic. It is the secretion of sebum onto the skin of the face and scalp that can become a problem for teenagers and older women alike as the face looks shiny, make-up runs, the presence of surface oil can cause blocked pores which attract dirt (blackheads), and infection of the ducts by microorganisms can produce pimples or acne.

Thorough cleansing of the skin is of vital importance - without stripping the skin of its protective mantle, which maintains the natural pH balance. It should be carried out, several times a day, using aromatic waters (gels) will prevent a buildup of sebum, on the skin's surface. Facial steaming and the use of clay masks can be very helpful in keeping the complexion clear and blemish free, and should include one of the following essential oils- Lemon, Geranium, Lavender, Bergamot (FCF), Juniper berry, Petit Grain, Neroli & Rosemary.

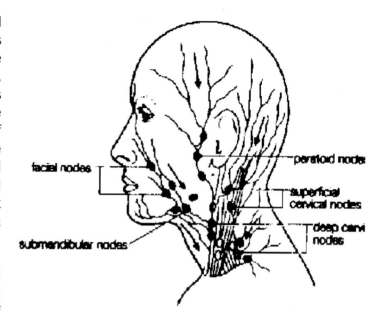

Cleansing with aromatic waters (gels) and using an aromatic facial steam bring the skin into contact with a very small amount of essential oil, which has beneficial results, but to treat a blemished complexion, it is necessary to apply a stronger concentration of essential oils in a light fatty oil base. The reason to use, a fatty oil on an already greasy skin, is firstly all fatty oils are not very greasy, secondly essential oils are far too concentrated to be used neat, and must always be diluted before applying to the skin and as essential oils dissolve in fatty acids, the preferred medium is fatty oil. Another reason is that fatty oils contain acids in much the same way as the skin and we know that essential oils dissolve into the oil secreted by the sebaceous glands. When an essential oil such as Lavender is massaged into the face, its antiseptic properties seep down into the deep layers of the skin to kill the bacteria, thus protecting and healing the skin and preventing infection.

* A simple recipe for a nightly cleansing massage is 2 drops of any one of the aforesaid essential oils plus 1 teaspoonful (5 Ml.) of good quality light fatty oil. Take care to remove all the traces of the oil from the face with a tissue or with cotton wool.

*or Add 3 drops each of Lemon, Rosemary, Petit and Lavender to 2 tablespoons (30 ml,) of light carrier oil such as grape seed, sweet almond or olive with avocado (for penetration) Massage gently all over and remove all the traces of the oil from the face with moist cotton swab, you'll be able to see all the dirt and grime.

* **Facial Steaming**- Spotty and greasy skins will benefit most from a facial steam once or twice a week incorporating a healing, antiseptic essential oils such as Tea tree, Geranium, Juniper berry or Lavender (only 3-5 drops in a bowl of steaming hot water), young problem skins also benefit from a facial steam once or twice a week, alternating with a face mask on other nights.

* A good toner/cleanser for greasy or combination skin is to mix 5 drops each of Petit grain, Juniper, Lavender and Geranium with 25 ml vodka and 75 ml orange flower water/ rose water. Let it stand for up to a month then filter. Use it for facial cleansing twice daily.

*After thorough cleansing you can nourish and moisturize face with rejuvenating massage oil containing any three to five of essential oils like- Lavender, Frankincense, Geranium, Sandalwood, Roman Chamomile or Juniper berry total 15 drops in two table spoon (30 ml.) of nourishing base oils like, Jojoba, sweet almond, Evening Primrose, Wheat germ. You can also make a combination of base oils to make your formulation more effective. This nourishing combination can be used once or twice daily preferably on moist skin after wash.

* An excellent basic purifying and rejuvenating face mask for greasy skin can be made by mixing 2 tablespoons green clay, 2 tablespoons cornflower, 1 egg yolk, 1 teaspoon evening primrose oil with 1 drop each of Rosemary and Lavender. Leave on the skin for 15 minutes then rinse off with cool water.

Dry & Dehydrated Skin- Dry skin becomes wrinkled more easily than greasy skin and needs to be moisturized regularly, especially when exposed to the effects of environment like by climate or too much sun or cold.

There are many essential oils which when blended together and incorporated into fatty base oil, make wonderful massage oils. We can create a blend to feed, regularize, moisturize, rejuvenate aging skin or bring antiseptic healing powers to troubled skin.

★ A good toner/cleanser for dry skin can be made by adding 5 drops each of Lemon, Lavender, Petit and Geranium to 100 ml rose water, letting it stand for up to a month before filtering.

★ Facial Steaming is also beneficial for dry skin incorporating healing, antiseptic essential oils such as sandal, lavender (only 3 drops in a bowl of hot water) once in a fortnight to be followed with moisturizer.

★ A moisturizing treatment for dry skin can be made by adding 5 drops each of lavender, geranium and sandal to 75 ml rose water, letting it stand for up to a month before filtering. Then add 25 ml glycerine and shake well. To be used twice daily.

★ For moisturizing dry sensitive skin, it is important to avoid all possible irritants and to use only the gentlest oils- Roman chamomile, Lavender, Sandal, Vertivert and Rose are the best choice. Add 7-8 drops of any of the above oils or a combination of 3-5 oils to 1 tablespoon (15 Ml.) combination of jojoba, sweet Almond or peach kernel oil or anti-allergic cream or lotion for daily use.

★ An excellent basic purifying and rejuvenating face mask for dry and sensitive skin can made by mixing 2 tablespoons of green clay, 2 teaspoons cornflower, 1 egg yolk, 1 teaspoon evening primrose oil (or almond oil) with 1 drop each of Geranium and Sandal. Leave on the skin for 15 minutes then rinse off, with cool water.

Aging Skin, Thread Veins & Wrinkles

There are two kinds of aging- one is INTRINSIC or CHRONOLOGICAL AGING, which is inevitable because of our body cell's potential for multiplying, but limited life expectancy. The body's own mechanisms control this, with things like hormones, growth factors and vitamins. Besides day to day physical, mental, emotional stresses also play a major role. Just as night follows the day, the passage of time means that it is inevitable that we will get older.

EXTRINSIC AGING- is mainly due to environmental factors like excess exposure to the sun. It can also be called photo intrinsic or active aging. Life style also affects aging.

As the skin gets older, cell division slows down and the skin becomes drier because of the reduced activity of the skin's oil glands. The slowing down of cell division means that the various organs in the skin work less efficiently. The inner dermis network of collagen and elastic fibers that give the skin its plain contours, suppleness and firmness begins to alter, losing its tension and plumpness and wrinkles form. The outer layer of skin cells, the epidermis also becomes thinner, resulting in the flat lifeless appearance of older skin.

Nothing can stop this natural process, but massage with essential oils can do more than most potions to slow down the effects. Essential oils encourage the skin cells to regenerate more efficiently and help the skin to lubricate itself, keeping it supple and less prone to wrinkling.

★ Regular use of facial oil containing cytophylactic oils (those that stimulate new cell growth and prevent wrinkles) is vital. They are Lavender, Geranium, Neroli, Frankicense, Sandal, Roman Chamomile, Rose and Palmarosa. Add 7-8 drops of the combination of any three of these oils to 1 tablespoon (15ml) of Jojoba or wheatgerm oil, for gentle application, especially to the area around the eyes before retiring.

★ A good basic blend for the face and neck is as follows 1 tablespoon (15 ml) Jojoba oil, 1 teaspoon (5ml) Wheat germ oil, 1 table spoon (15 ml) 6 drops of lavender, 4 drops of geranium, 3 drops of frankincense and 2 drops sandalwood oil.

★ Thread veins and broken capillaries are best treated using aforesaid facial oil with the addition of 1 drops of German Chamomile or rose oil.

★ A face mask made by mixing 2 tablespoons green clay, 2 teaspoons runny honey, 1 teaspoon water and 4 drops of rose oil, used once a week, helps rejuvenation. You may also add 2 drops of Lavender and 1 drop of Geranium to enhance the effect.

FRICTION MASSAGE FOR REJUVENATION

Most beauticians insist that facial massage should be of lightest possible strokes for fear of stretching the delicate tissues of the skin. It's true in the case of sensitive skin or acne or skin with broken veins - as in these cases skin should be handled with gentle care. But in case of normal, dry or aging skin, friction massage with selected essential oils blend has many benefits, it tones the underlying muscles, keeping them in good shape; it nourishes the skin by bringing blood to the surface, thereby allowing dietary nutrients available for cell renewal. It also rubs away dead skin cells helping to make the complexion look lighter and more youthful.

Secure hair back from forehead and apply the massage oil blend from hairline to the chin, work on one section of the face at a time. Tense the muscles (as a man does when shaving) so that the skin is not stretched. Starting with one section (say the left cheek) press and rotate the skin and underlying muscles, using the first three fingers of the left hand. Feel for any sore areas, and gently but firmly massage those areas until the skin begins to feel hot. Next, put your right thumb inside your mouth so that the pad of the thumb is pressing against the inside of the cheek. Squeeze flesh between thumb and fingers and move the thumb in tiny circular movements so that all of the flesh inside the cheek has been massaged. Repeat the movements on the right side of the face. Next, place your palms of hands on the cheeks and with facial muscles tensed; buff the cheeks with circular movements. Massage of the forehead follows and in order to tense the muscles it is simple to close the eyes tightly, and then to buff the skin with palm of the hand. Begin in the centre of the forehead and with a circular motion work outwards towards the temples. Before massaging the chin, place the lips together so that the lips are visible (as woman does to spread lipstick evenly after application) and with the palm of the hands,

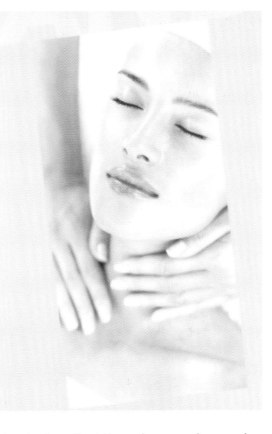

buff the skin. Move the mouth (again as a man does while shaving) so that there is enough muscles tension and massage in this way around to the mouth, so that tiny lines are encouraged to disappear.

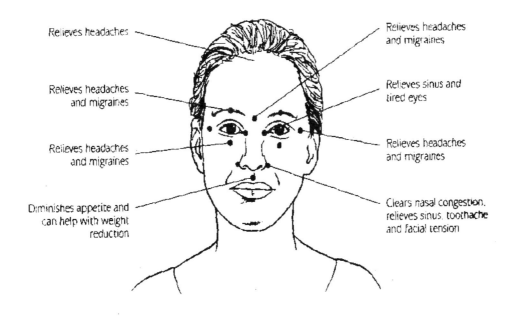

Relieves headaches

Relieves headaches and migraines

Relieves headaches and migraines

Diminishes appetite and can help with weight reduction

Relieves headaches and migraines

Relieves sinus and tired eyes

Relieves headaches and migraines

Clears nasal congestion, relieves sinus, toothache and facial tension

Major accupressure points on the face and their benefits

DOUBLE CHIN-

Double chin can be greatly hewed by massaging skin with the following blend:

To a 30 ml. bottle add:
3 drops Lemon grass oil
3 drops Grape fruit oil
3 drops Lavender oil
3 drops Cypress oil
3 drops Orange oil
15 ml. Jojoba oil
15 ml. White carrier oil

Though this lemongrass is very powerful and not used on face normally as it can irritate the delicate skin, however it has a remarkable ability, to decongest the tissues by burning up toxins in the connective tissue, chin is an area where fat can accumulate easily and where toxins can lodge.

Apply the above blend to the underside of the chin and tilt back so that the skin of the neck is taut. Using only the tips of the first two fingers of each hand, slide the fingertips along jaw-line until they reach the angle of the jaw. Repeat several times. Position the same fingers under jawbone in the centre of the chin and gently stroke the "double chin", drawing the fingers down the neck toward the cervical lymph nodes. Continue this gentle stroking of the under-chin area and be sensitive to any lumps and bumps that may be under the skin's surface. Gently massage these toxic and stagnant spots to encourage them to disperse and immediately after working on this area, spend a few moments massaging the lymph nodes involved with the drainage of fats and toxins from the head and neck.

If the skin under the chin is very loose and flabby replace lemongrass oil by vertivert oil in the aforesaid blend and massage the area, as vertivert oil has the ability to attract and retain moisture in the underlying tissues of the skin, making the flesh look plumper.

ACNE (PIMPLES OR SPOTS)

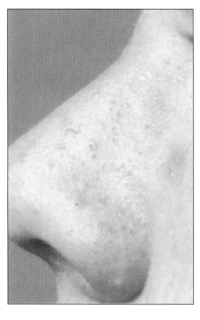

Acne is a condition in which the skin of the face and sometimes at the neck, shoulders, chest and back is covered to a greater or lesser extent with pimples, blackheads, whiteheads and boils. Acne usually results from hormonal imbalance or an incorrect diet or both being the factors that affect the production of sebum. In case of acne due to hormonal disturbance, taking Evening primrose oil 1 teaspoonful orally on daily basis for three months helps a great deal.

A variety of factors including too frequent washing, an unhealthy diet; hormonal imbalance and stress may affect the production of sebum and sweat, causing too much or too little to be secreted, with consequent greasy or dry skin. The typical onset of acne in adolescence is related to the increased activity of the glands, including the sebaceous glands.

Most of the oil gets into pores, when the surface pores are clogged with sebaceous gland secretions & keratin, and when so much extra oil is being secreted that it backs up into the ducts, the result is the formation of the skin blemishes, characteristic of acne.

The blackheads are dark not because they are dirty but because the fatty material in the clogged pore is oxidized and discolored by the air that reaches it, when this substance is infected by bacteria, it turns into a pimple. Under no circumstances should pimples be picked or squeezed, because the pressure can rupture the surrounding membrane and spread the infection further.

Treatment-

Life-style- Gentle ultra-violet rays can, greatly relieve acne so take every opportunity you can to go out in the sun, but do not over expose the skin.

Diet- Should incorporate healthy balanced diet, avoiding spicy and fatty foods, in particular dairy products. Diet should include plenty of other sources of protein and calcium rich food. Eat plenty of fresh fruits and green vegetables. Drink up to four pints of mineral water daily.

Essential oils- That regulate sebum production and purify the blood include Juniper berry, Lemon, cypress and Geranium. Tea tree, Lavender, Palmarosa and Geranium are antiseptic and healing, while German chamomile and Petitgrain help to reduce inflamation.

★ Apply an aromatic flower water as a toner/cleanser to the skin, morning and evening. To prepare mix 25 ml cider vinegar, 75 ml rose water with 5 drops each of Lemon, Geranium, Tea tree and Lavender. Let it mature for up to a month, and then filter before use with coffee filter paper. (It is better to make a batch in one go only).

★ Use a light facial oil containing two teaspoons Grape seed oil, 1 teaspoon wheat germ oil , and 1 teaspoon of Jojoba oil, in the base and add 3 drops each of Tea tree, Juniper, Geranium and Lavender. Apply gently every night after washing face on moist skin, it will also help clearing acne scars.

★ Individual pimples can be dabbed with neat Lavender and Tea tree (check sensitization first).

★ A good facial mask can be made by mixing 2 tablespoons of green clay or kaolin. 2 teaspoon of yoghurt or rose water with 2 drops each of juniper, geranium and cypress.

★ To unclog the pores of the skin, put 3 drops each of Petit grain and Geranium in a bowl of steaming water as facial steam. Putting pine needle oil mixed with water on the stove when having sauna has a similar effect on the whole body.

Emergency Pimples Treatment- Pimples should never be squeezed when they are small red bumps, because at this stage there is nothing to remove and result is only bruising of the tissues. However, when a pimple has come to a head, you have a choice of whether to dab it with neat Lavender and Tea tree or in case of emergency squeeze the spot. Though it is not recommended still if carried out carefully you can get rid of the waste material and white head in the pimple. If the later course of action is chosen because of circumstances like wedding or a social occasion, then very carefully set about removing as under.

A sharp needle should be sterilized by first wiping with a piece of cotton wool moistened with one drop of lavender. Gently prick the spot with the needle- not downward into the spot, but sideways so that the tip of the needle is parallel with the face. With clean cotton wool apply sufficient pressure to discharge the accumulated debris (a mixture of bacteria and dead lymph cells) and finally, dab the area with one of the antiseptic oils Lavender, Tea tree, Juniper, Lemon, Palmarosa or Bergamot. It may sting for a few seconds but it will prevent the spread of infection. And no make up for 24 hours.

An alternate to squeezing is to take facial steam at the first signs of a spot. The hot, moist vapors combined with antiseptic and healing aromas promote elimination through the skin and help to unblock the clogged pores- often the cause of blackheads and spots (pimples).

The Eyes

It is said that eyes are the windows to the soul. Whether it's true or not they are still the most expressive features- and should be prepared and cared for. The best eye treatment of all is a "good night sleep". But, with the kind of lifestyle we all have, have late nights, looking at TV/computer screens most of the time, spending time around smokers or in polluted air or have allergies or mascara not removed or make up remover going in the eyes and all that- results into your "windows" going to look puffy, bloodshot, irritated or have dark circles beneath them. They may even sting and tear.

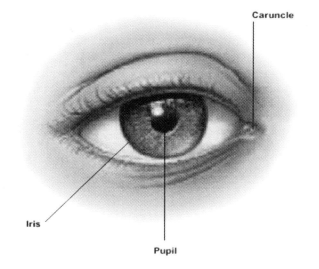

For a Night Time Eye Moisturizer- On a damp freshly cleansed face apply a few drops of Jojoba, Grape seed, Sweet almond or Evening Primrose oil-mix together with your ring finger then gently pat the oil around (not directly on) the eye in the following fashion:
Begin at the outer corner and slowly move beneath your eye toward the inner corner, then onto the very upper portion of the lid and back out to the outer corner.

Do this several times, and then pat of any excess oil. Try to leave a thin film of oil on the skin. The oil should not be applied directly on the lids and lashes. If the oil gets into the eye, it could clog the tear ducts and cause puffiness (which we are trying to avoid). The delicate eye area will draw the moisture it needs from the surrounding moisturized tissue.

You can also use an aromatic eye compress using Lavender aromatic water (prepare by adding 10 drops lavender oil in 200 ml. spring water - shake well) to soothe irritated, puffy eyes. A piece of cotton pad is saturated with lavender aromatic water, remove excess by squeezing before applying the pad to the eyes. Lie down for at least ten minutes whilst the compress is in place. Another alternative to this compress is thin slices of cold cucumber or potato.

Crow's Feet- To treat wrinkles of the delicate skin around the eye and tighten the skin apply an egg's white face mask add Rose or Geranium oil to the mask. Whisk the egg white in a small bowl and when frothy add 2 drops of Rose or Geranium oil. Mix for a few seconds more and apply to the skin immediately around the eye socket. Upper eyelids and eyebrows may be included in this tightening mask. Allow to dry and rinse off with wet cotton pads. Whilst skin is still damp, apply a little of Wheat germ oil and Jojoba oil blend and gently pat into the skin at outer edges of eyes.

Thin Eyelashes and Eyebrows- When eyelashes become thin because of constant wearing of mascara, they should be given a holiday from mascara and instead be treated with coating of Jojoba oil. Eyelashes, like hair on our head, are dead and therefore apply this blend with mascara applicator and also massage a little on to the eyelids, where the lashes spring forth. The skin surrounding the eye is very sensitive and feeding of the eyelashes should not be repeated too frequently. Application, once a week is ample.

The condition of eyebrows specially thin & straggly can also be improved by rubbing a little jojoba oil along their length.

Lips- Our lips, unlike the rest of our skin, do not contain any sebaceous glands (oil glands) or sweat glands to keep them moisturized and lubricated. The lipsticks used on the lips besides beautifying should also prevent them from drying and cracking, but many of the lipstick brands instead of, tend to dry lips. That can make the lips to flake and peel and make them unsightly.
Dry lips may also occur, when we are unavoidably outside on a windy day or when we have too much sun on our face. However, dry lips also denote that we are not drinking enough water.

You can prepare a protective lip balm as under:

2 teaspoons (10ml) bees wax,   5 teaspoons (25ml) jojoba oil
1 teaspoon (5ml) Avacado oil,   1 teaspoons (5ml) Honey
5 drops essential oil of Geranium, Lavender and sandal

This is good for everyone; even children. Use- as desired
Preparation time- 20-30 minutes
Mix with: Spoon
Store: Small glass or plastic lip balm jars
Yield: Approximately 1 1/3 ounce (40ml)
Suitable: For chapped/ dry lips can double as cuticle cream

Method of preparation- Melt together the oil and beeswax, in a small saucepan over low heat, or in double boiler just until wax is melted. Use larger amount of oil for thinner, glossier consistency. Remove from heat. Add honey and blend mixture thoroughly. Stir mixture occasionally as it cools to prevent separation. When the mixture is almost cooled, add the essential oils and stir thoroughly. This lip balm should have the consistency of paste wax when ready.

Head & Hair Care

Healthy Hair: Our hair is only a collection of individual hairs– approximately 250000, each one is deep rooted in the scalp, and just as dependent on good nutrition as the skin or any other part of our body. Hair originates & tiny sacs or follicles deep in the dermis layer of skin tissue. The part of the hair below the skin surface is the root; the part above is the shaft. Hair follicles are closely connected to the sebaceous glands, which secrete oil to the scalp and give hair its natural sheen. Hair grows at the rate of 1 centimeter per month, although some people's hair grow faster or slower than the average. Healthy growth of hair depends a lot on the diet. Healthy diet leads to healthy hair.

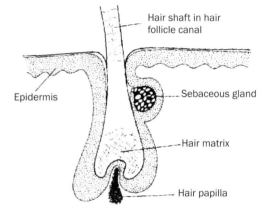

Hair is a complex cellular structure. The structural form is basically the same, each strand, no matter how fine it may look, consists of three layers. The outer layer or cuticle is made up of overlapping scales which protect the inner layers. The next layer or the cortex is made up of long thin cells and is the most important, for it gives the hair its elastic resilience and contains the pigment which provides the coloring. The innermost layer or medulla is spongy tissue and the cells sometimes contain granules of color pigment.

The part of the hair visible above the skin is the SHAFT and the part beneath is the root. The root is not a single entity, as it is enclosed in a sac called hair follicle, and at the base of this is a tiny hair nodule called the papilla, which is the store house for the nourishment of hair strand. Interlinked to the follicles are sacs containing sebum which lubricates the hair and gives it gloss and suppleness. An under active or blocked sebaceous gland means dry hair, an over active one means oily hair.

We are inclined to forget that healthy hair is a part of a healthy body, and directly affected by physical metabolism and emotional balance. Its texture may be determined by genes but its strength and condition are determined by what it is fed. A high protein diet with lots of fresh fruits and vegetables is good for hair. Foods containing vitamins of the B complex are essential. Also important, are vitamins A and C, and the minerals of iron, iodine, and copper are the most beneficial, and lack of iodine can be most detrimental.

Like Skin, hair can be DRY, OILY or BALANCED. The wonderful washablilty of hair is one of its main assets. The ritual of washing is the first and basic beauty routine as all hair types. Oily hair require washing every two to three days, while dry hair can be washed every 5 to 7 days. The rule is to wash when hair looks or feels dirty and the modern rule is wash often, wash lightly, use shampoo sparingly. Sometimes, even if diet is sensible and nutritious, we may not benefit from the nutrients, if our body is not absorbing enough vitamins and minerals from what we have eaten. Stress is one common reason why we sometimes fail to absorb sufficient goodness from our food. This is why, when someone is suffering badly from stress, their hair can start thinning and their skin may look as though they have suddenly "aged". Natural hair loss is between 50-100 hairs, more than that is considered abnormal.

Topically, there is much we can do to improve the condition of the scalp- the flower bed or the soil from which the hair blossoms. And just as we must feed the soil if we wish to produce beautiful roses, so it is with our scalp. Essential oils, when massaged into the scalp, will penetrate through the epidermis to the dermis and connective tissue where the hair bulb is rooted.

Useful oils- The perfect combination of external nutrients, for the scalp and hair, are the aromatherapy essential and base oils. While Rosemary and Ylang Ylang stimulate the scalp, Ylang Ylang and Cedar wood are balancing oils which will help to prevent further hair loss. Jojoba oil protects and contributes greatly to the process of cell renewal, therefore recommended as a base oil, even sweet almond is considered as a tonic for the scalp, for all types of hair.

Head & Hair Treatment

Massage- Gentle nightly massage of the scalp will relieve any tightness caused by stress. When stressed our muscles tense up causing, amongst other problems headaches and nausea. But beyond the noticeable physical symptoms, tension is also responsible for preventing the normal circulation of blood and lymph, sebum and other nutrients. In effect, if we are really stressed out, we can literally be starving our hair to death. Massaging the head will dispel tension caused by stress, whether emotional, mental or environmental, by relaxing the scalp and allowing the circulation of blood, lymph and sebum. Besides essential oils diluted in jojoba are used for the purpose of massage enhancing the effect of massage by providing external nutrients thereby prevent the hair loss and improving the health of the scalp.

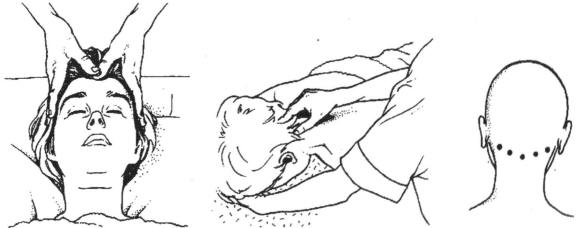

* You can choose any of the following formulations as per the hair type:

For dry, lack luster hair	For excess grease	For normal hair
2 drops of Rosemary oil	2drops of Juniper oil	2 drops of Palmarosa Oil
2 drops of Lavender oil	2 drops of Lemon oil	2 drops Lemon oil
2 drops of Cedar wood oil	2 drops of Rosemary oil	2 drops Rosemary oil
2 drops of patchouli oil	2 drops Cedarwood oil	2 drops Ylang Ylang oil
4 teaspoons of jojoba oil	2 teaspoons jojoba oil	2 teaspoon Jojoba oil
1 Teaspoon Wheat germ oil	3 Teaspoon Grapeseed oil	3 teaspoon Seasme oil

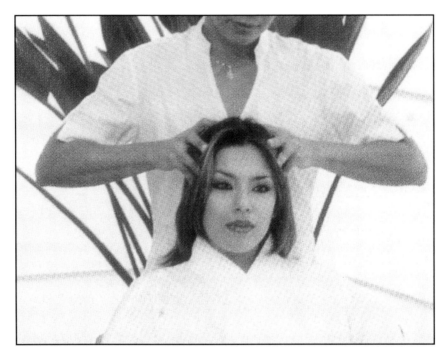

*A few drops (approximately 1 per cent) of an essential oil suited to your hair type can be added to your shampoo it is always better to use a mild or PH neutral shampoo which does not strip the hair of its protective acid mantle. For greasy hair, use Rosemary and Lemon, for dry hair use Patchouli or Cedar wood, for normal dark hair rosemary and Ylang Ylang oil.

*A good rinse for all hair types is- to add 5 drops of Rosemary or Ylang Ylang essential oils to 1 tablespoon cider vinegar using it for the final rinse, it will also help to remove soap/ shampoo chemicals residue and restore the pH balance of the scalp.

Dandruff

Dandruff may take the form of fine, dry powdery flakes or coarse, waxy scales that stick to the hair and scalp causing intense irritation. Resist the temptation to scratch your head with the latter type of dandruff, since this may cause bleeding and infection. In case the facial skin becomes oily and pimples/spots develop on forehead, wash hair frequently and choose a hair style that keeps the hair off the forehead. Sometimes this condition can easily be confused with either eczema or psoriasis of the scalp, so it is important to obtain an accurate diagnosis from a trichologist.

Treatment

Lifestyle and Diet- In case of oily scaling dandruff, wash your hair frequently, using a mild shampoo. Use plenty of exercise, outdoors in the fresh air, avoid spicy food and dairy products. Dry dandruff is often stress related.

Application- Depending on the type of scalp choose any of the recipe

For dry flaking scalp -   3 drops of Lavender
  3 drops of Geranium oil
  6 drops of Rosemary oil
  3 drops Tea tree oil
  4 drops Cedar wood oil
  5-6 teaspoons of Carrier oil

For oily scaling scalp -

5 drops of Atlas Cedarwood oil
5 drops of Rosemary oil
5 drops of Lemon oil
5 drops Juniper Berry oil
5-6 teaspoon of Carrier oil or vodka.

These blends should be massaged in the scalp and left for two hours or over-night. Shampoo and rinse thoroughly, make up the final rinse by adding the same blend of essential oils to jug of water. Stir well before using. Repeat treatment every alternate day decreasing to twice a week.

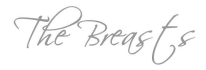

The Breasts

> **The Problems-** *Sagging breasts, Fibrocystic (lumpiness) breasts, too large or too small, stretch marks and blemishes.*
>
> **The Causes-** *Loss of elasticity, gravity, genetics. Poor circulation, hormonal imbalances, Rapid weight gain or loss.*
>
> **The Solutions-** *Skin brushing while bathing, massage and chest packs.*

The breasts are the ultimate symbol of womanly beauty. No more than a mass of adipose tissue until hormonally changed into a milk producing machine, although coveted objects of adornment, are often neglected in terms of physical care, merely to be crammed into bras, Basques and bodies- completely taken for granted. Like the rest of the body, the breasts contain connective tissues which siphon off toxins and infections, and muscle fiber, which can be damaged either by being stretched or by constantly under tension. Massage of the breasts with aromatic oils can help to keep the breasts not only in good shape but also in good health too.

What are fibrocystic breasts?

Fibrocystic breasts are characterized by lumpiness and unusual discomfort in one or both breasts. The condition is very common and benign, meaning that fibrocystic breasts are not malignant (cancerous). Fibrocystic breast disease (FBD), now referred to as fibrocystic changes or fibrocystic breast condition. It is the most common cause of "lumpy breasts" in women and affects more than 60% of women. The condition primarily affects women between the ages of 30 and 50 and tends to become less of a problem after menopause.

What causes fibrocystic breasts?

Fibrocystic breast condition involves the glandular breast tissue. The sole known biologic function of these glands is the production, or secretion, of milk. Occupying a major portion of the breast, the glandular tissue is surrounded by fatty tissue and support elements. The glandular tissue is composed of different types of cells: (1) clusters of secretary cells (cells that produce milk) that are connected to the milk ducts (tiny tubes); and (2) the cells that line the surfaces of the secretary cells, called the epithelial cells.

The most significant contributing factor to fibrocystic breast condition is a woman's normal hormonal changes during her monthly cycle. Many hormonal changes occur as a woman's body prepares each month for a possible pregnancy. The most important of these hormones are estrogen and progesterone. These two hormones directly affect the breast tissues by causing cells to grow and multiply.

The same cyclical hormones that prepare the glandular tissue in the breast for the possibility of milk production (lactation) are also responsible for a woman's menstrual period. However, there is a major difference between what happens in the breast and uterus. In the uterus (the womb), these hormones promote the growth and multiplication of the cells lining the uterus. If pregnancy does not occur, this uterine lining is sloughed off and discharged from a woman's body during menstruation.

In the breast, these same hormones stimulate the growth of breast glandular tissue and increase the activity of blood vessels, cell metabolism, and supporting tissue. All this activity may contribute to the feeling of breast fullness and fluid retention that women commonly experience before their menstrual period.

When the monthly cycle is over, however, these stimulated breast cells cannot simply slough away and pass out of the body like the lining of the uterus. Instead, many of these breast cells undergo a process of programmed cell death, called apoptosis. During apoptosis, enzymes are activated that start digesting cells from within. These cells break down and the resulting cellular fragments are then further broken down by scavenger cells (inflammatory cells) and nearby glandular cells.

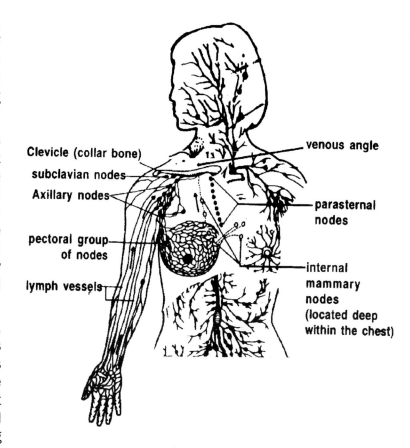

Clevicle (collar bone)
subclavian nodes
Axillary nodes
pectoral group of nodes
lymph vessels
venous angle
parasternal nodes
internal mammary nodes (located deep within the chest)

During this process, the fragments of broken cells and the inflammation may lead to scarring (fibrosis) that damages the ducts and the clusters (lobules) of glandular tissue within the breast. The inflammatory cells and some of the breakdown fragments may release hormonelike substances that in turn act on the nearby glandular, ductal, and structural support cells. The amount of cellular breakdown products, the degree of inflammation, and the efficiency of the cellular cleanup process in the breast vary from woman to woman. These factors may also fluctuate from month to month in an individual woman. They may even vary in different areas of the same breast in a woman.

Fibrocystic breast condition is said to primarily affect women age 30 and older. The reason for this is that the condition likely results from a cumulative process of repeated monthly hormonal cycles and the accumulation of fluid, cells, and cellular debris within the breast. The process starts with puberty and continues through menopause. After menopause, fibrocystic breast condition becomes less of a problem. Out of my experience of healing work, I have observed that our blocked emotions affect two of our Chakras the most- Sacral and heart. In case of sacral chakra blockage, due to emotional issues, lymphatics (primarily inguinal nodes) may get blocked and become sore, affecting ovulation, menstrual cycle (irregular or painful) sometime leading to uterine fibroids. When heart chakra is blocked because of painful emotions like anguish, it affects auxiliary nodes and circulation around the breast area, can also be one of the causes for fibrocystic breast conditions.

Treatment for Fibrocystic Breast condition

I have observed positive results on breast lumps by aroma oils massage coupled with Evening Primrose oil ingestion. Recommended dosage is 5 ml (1 teaspoon) of pure evening primrose oil, initially for 3 to 6 months. (refer to the chapter on evening primrose oil in the book).Recommended essential oils are Juniper berry, Rose or Geranium, Clary Sage and Fennel seed oils. You can use 4 drops of each of these oils in two tablespoons (30 ml.) of a good base oil. To be massaged twice daily all around the breast termination in the arm pits.

Sagging Breasts with Stretch Marks

When there is a sudden weight gain or loss, the skin sometimes scars, leaving a constant reminder of weight change in the form of tiny silver lines. Stretch marks cannot vanish in just two to three weeks as it takes far longer than that for new skin to grow, but it is possible to reduce the visible scarring over a period of time. Just by massaging the breasts with suitable essential oil blend and by increasing the elasticity of the skin, the effect of the stretch-marks will lessen and improve the breast tone.

<u>Skin Brushing-</u> As a measure of self-help to take care of breasts, once a week skin brushing is important. For skin brushing, take a nail brush and without using much pressure, run the bristles from the breast bone out to the arm pit. Brush across the entire breast, always in the direction of the armpits where the auxiliary lymph nodes are housed. Lifting up one arm, brush the underside of the upper arm, towards the armpit and then brush the armpit itself. Underneath this area of skin, which has made a huge amount of money for perfumes & deodorant industry, lies a cluster of lymph nodes, vitally placed to drain lymph from the arms and breasts (see figure), You can even use your hand to massage yourself everyday while taking your shower and when you remove your bra. Use your knuckles to knead the area of armpits to decongest the auxiliary nodes.

<u>Breast Massage-</u> The massage techniques are the same for every woman, the only difference being the blend of the oils used. For regular massage the following blend is most suitable

2 drops Geranium oil
2 drops Lavender oil
1 drop Vertiver oil
1 drop Cypress oil
In 4 teaspoons of suitable carrier oil.

For women who feel their breasts are too small and would try to increase their size, the following blend will be most suitable

2 drops Geranium oil
3 drops Vertivert oil
2 drops Lavender oil

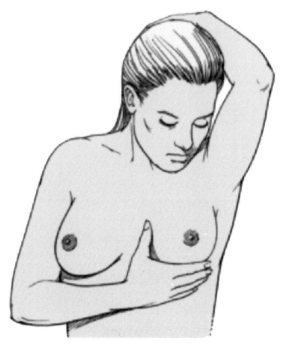

2 drops Clary Sage oil
In 4 teaspoons of suitable Carrier oil.

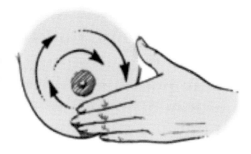

Whichever blend is chosen, and whether or not a change in size is achieved, massage oil will definitely improve the muscle tone of the breasts and perk up the sagging breasts. The feel of skin will become silky and smooth, and the general health of the breasts will improve.

During the massage the lymph nodes get massaged, taking away toxins and dead matter from the mammary glands and bring a fresh supply of lymph containing lymphocytes to recognize and kill unwanted organisms such as bacteria and viruses, boosting immune system.

Chest Pack-

Sometimes the skin in the centre of the chest (from just above the cleavage to the base of the neck) become spotty, which is the last thing wanted by anybody. Just as a face pack constantly refreshes and revitalizes the skin, so does a chest pack. Follow it after brast massage.

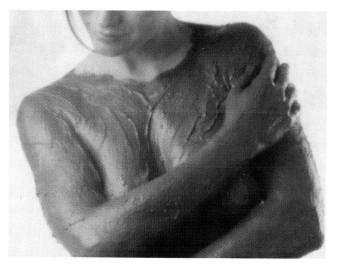

To prepare a chest pack, take the following
2 table spoon Green Clay
2 tablespoons Kaolin
2 teaspoons water
2 drops Myrtle oil or Geranium oil.

Mix and add 1 teaspoon Jojoba oil and spread across the chest. After applying the mask, it is advisable to lie down for approximately 15 minutes while the clay, dries up. Cover chest with a hand towel before getting up to clean to avoid dry clay flaking off. After cleaning, pat dry.

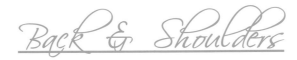

Back & Shoulders

The Problems- *Congested skin dotted with pimples, greasy skin with open pores, dull looking skin, tension in upper back & neck, stiffness in the shoulders.*

Causes- *Lack of movement (of skin and muscles), stagnation, emotional / mental stress, lack of air, improper diet, dehydration.*

Solutions- *Aromatic baths (cleaning with friction strip), skin brushing, back compress with body wrap, and massage.*

All the above problems respond to bathing with aromatic oils friction and skin brushing. Some of them like congested skin, greasy skin and dull looking skin- can be treated by a body wrap or back pack. For stiffness and tension in the neck and shoulders the best way is 'massage' starting from the center of neck, with gentle kneading, followed by massage and lymphatic drainage towards the arm pits.

Pimples or spots in the back are due to bacterial infection mostly a result of dandruff. Since all the essential oils are bactericidal their use in any form whether in bath, compress, as massage oil or body wrap- is very effective in tackling the condition.

Aromatic bath for Shoulders- Congested skin on the back can be stimulated and improve considerably only by taking an aromatic bath with 6-10 drops of either Lavender, Juniper, Geranium or Rosemary or combination of all. Alternatively a blend of 3 drops lavender, 2 drops Juniper and 3 drops of rosemary can be used.

For the greasy skin most suitable oils are Lemon, Juniper berry, Lavender, Rosemary, Geranium, and Petit grain.

For dry skin suitable oils are sandalwood, Patchouli, Lavender, Geranium or Frankincense.

Skin Brushing- While bathing to stimulate the skin in its efforts to eliminate unwanted matters and toxins is important. Skin brushing with a lufah or a brush will also serve the purpose just run the bristles along the upper arm from elbow to shoulders and from the crease of the elbow to the armpit, until entire skin surface is covered. Then brush across the shoulders and behind the neck up to the collar bone. Under the collar bone is a collection of lymph nodes which drain impurities away from the upper chest and neck. Women are particularly vulnerable to congestion around the shoulders because of the bra they have to wear 8 - 12 hours a day, which will definitely cause a certain amount of pressure; even slight pressure endured for a protracted period of time will have a negative effect.

Friction Rub- Back is an ideal site for elimination of body's toxins and waste products. A spotty back with white/ blackheads can be caused by a build- up sweat and sebum which has not been cleaned thoroughly.

The skin of the back can be scrubbed off with a friction strip or towel. Let the skin be soaked in aromatic bath waters for a while, before cleaning with friction.

Body Wrap- Body wrap, is a sort of wet pack, as called by naturopaths. It is the simplest and most effective way of decongesting the skin of the back and shoulders especially if massage is not possible. Half fill a hand basin with comfortably hot water; add 6 drops in total of Juniper berry, Lavender or Rosemary. Agitate the water to ensure that oils are fully dispersed and dip in a big enough cotton towel, wring out the excess water; spread the towel on the back and shoulder, ask somebody to put a sheet of plastic over the towel so that the heat of the towel is conserved. Relax for a while. You can use this treatment sitting or lying down position. This allows, to draw impurities out of the body in a simple relaxed way.

Aromatic Back Pack- Aromatic back pack is sort of messy but very helpful to refine skin of the upper back, especially between the shoulders where sebum can clog pores and spots accumulate.

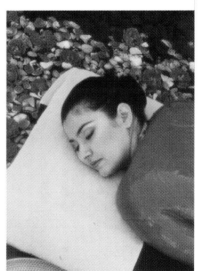

The oils effective for aromatic pack are- Bergamot, Lemon, Grape fruit, Lavender, Tea tree, Neroli, Juniperberry & geranium.

Take100 gms. Fuller's earth (Multani Mitti)/green clay.
Add sufficient water to make a fine paste.
Then add 5-6 drops of chosen essential oils.
Mix together and apply.

Let the pack be there for half an hour, then shower it off. It is preferable and easier to dispose of dry clay, instead of washing it down through the bathroom drain. The ultimate result of the back pack is a tingling clean and clear skin at the back.

Massage- The back massage with aromatic oil blends will mainly consist of effleurage with some kneading of the areas of tension. For a truly effective back massage, around 20 minutes are required. The following massage blends can be used -

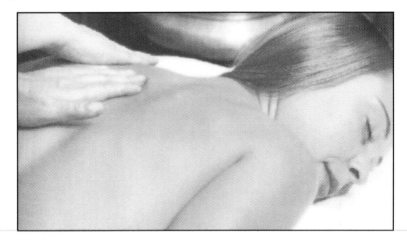

Relaxing Blend

3 drops Sandal
3 drops Lavender
2 drops Patchauli

15 ml Chosen carrier oil

Invigorating Blend

3 drops rosemary
2 drops Grape Fruit
3 drops Lemon Grass

15 ml Chosen carrier oil.

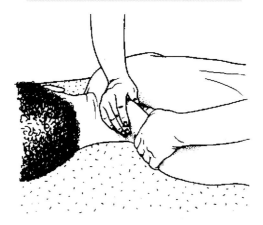
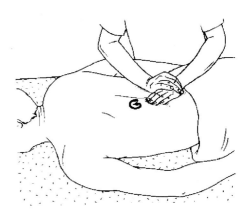

After the back massage, it is advisable to massage the points on the chest just above and below the clavicle as this is where the lymph drains into the blood stream. Nature really is incredible- she has positioned the main lymph drains on the front of the body where they can be reached easily. The main thoracic duct runs up the back in parallel with the spine and drains its lymph into the left venous angle. Lymph from the right side of the chest, face and head drains into the right venous angle. These points can be massaged at any time of the day. If you do not have access to massage just apply the aromatic oils to the shoulder and neck where tension is stored and stiffness is often registered.

Massaging, stroking and pressing different points around the neck, shoulders and upper back not only helps to feel better in short term but to function more effectively in the long run.

Tummy, Waist, And Abdomen

The Problems- *Excess fat, wrinkles, tension stored in the solar plexus.*

The Causes- *Fat deposits; toxic wastes, anxiety and stress.*

The Solutions- *Aromatic bath, skin brushing; massage.*

Tummy and Waist

The tummy is often the first place where we notice an increase in weight or increase in girth. When skirts no longer fit and trousers will not zip up, we know that we have amassed excess fat. But why does fat accumulate so easily around the waist?

One reason may be that there are very few lymph nodes on the front of the torso. From the navel upwards, the lymph vessels take fluids and drain them to the auxiliary nodes under the arms, and from the navel downwards, the lymph drains to the inguinal nodes in the groin. Because there are no lymph nodes actually at the waist, it is easy for cells to become crammed full of fat. By encouraging the flow of lymph to the nodes which will filter and brea⁀ down the fat deposits, we can hel⌐ control, the size of our waists. Fror the inguinal nodes lymph flows t⌐ the intestinal and lumber trunk⌐ (which also drain fluid from the entire abdominal cavity) into the cisterna chyli, which lies deep in the body, next to the vertebrae.

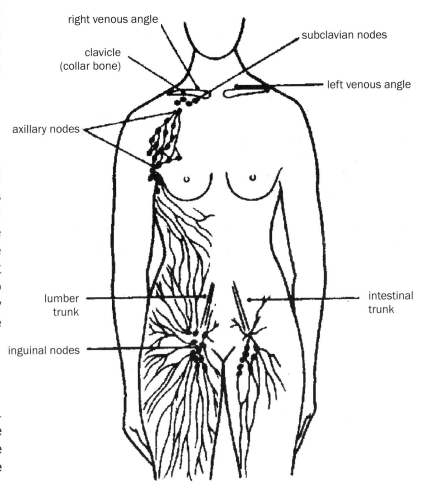

right venous angle

subclavian nodes

clavicle (collar bone)

left venous angle

axillary nodes

lumber trunk

intestinal trunk

inguinal nodes

From the cisterna chyli, which is on a level with the navel, but deeper in the body, the lymph flows into the thoracic duct and travels up the body almost parallel with the spine before dividing into two parts at the level of the heart. The left fork drains into the left venous angle, a large vein sited above the left collarbone. Also draining into this vein is lymph from the left side of the face, head, chest and arm. Lymph from the right side of the head, face, chest and arm drains into the right lymphatic duct at the right venous angle above the right collar bone.

Aromatic Baths-

Bath with oils such as juniper, orange which aid in the dispersal of unwanted fats and fluids, or bath in essences which are hyper-aemic (such as myrtle) and bring fresh blood to the skin's surface. This helps to tone and firm the tummy as fresh blood brings with it nutrients to feed the skin. Lymphatic movement is also stimulated, allowing fats to be broken down and carried away from the site, eventually to be expelled from the body. Many fats are recycled by the body simply because the liver is not able to cope up with large quantities.

Stress release is of great importance when we are endeavoring to get rid of the unwanted layers of fat. Stress affects people in different ways, and for some people too much stress can interfere with the efficient metabolism of the body allowing a build-up of fatty deposits. It also makes the solar plexus tight with all bottled up stress and anxieties. It is useful to add anti-stress oils to the bath, such as geranium, Lavender and Rose.

Skin Brushing-

Skin brushing of the abdomen is very effective because the concentration of the adipose fat makes it difficult for essential oils to penetrate. Skin brushing stimulates the movement of the fat and lymph encourages drainage of unwanted toxins as well as the increased absorption of essential oils. If you intend to massage the tummy and waist later, skin brush the whole of the abdomen- the abdomen is the area from the diaphragm to the floor of the pelvis- as it will prepare the skin for the essential oil blends.

Take a brush and stroke from the navel downwards to the 'knickers line", brushing the skin across the inguinal nodes at the top of the legs. Then brush from the navel upwards to the diaphragm, and skirting around the breasts, sweep up to the auxiliary nodes at the armpit.

Massage of Tummy and Waist

Massage of tummy and waist can help to eliminate toxins, break up fatty deposits and encourage their dispersal, toning up the skin and underlying muscle so that wrinkles are reduced. If the flesh hurts when pinched between the thumb and fingers, this could indicate that the tissues are home to stagnant wastes so choose the lemongrass blend containing
    5 drops of Lemon grass.
    8 drops of Grapefruit oil.
    5 drops of Lemon
    Added to 30 ml of Chosen carrier oil having at least 25% jojoba oil and 10 % Avocado Oil

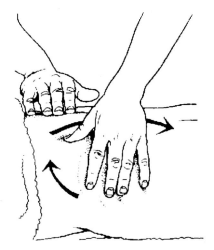 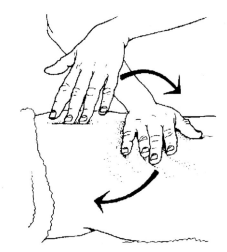

Choose the following juniper blend if you are prone to occasional water retention and the unwanted inches around your waist contain not only fatty tissue but also excess fluid.

You can also prepare a juniper blend with:

    5 drops of Juniper Berry oil
    5 drops Grape Fruit oil
    5 drops Orange oil
    5 drops fennel seed oil
    30 ml special Carrier oils as mentioned above.

Cling Film Wrap- An effective, though not permanent way to whittle away the waist is to give yourself a Cling film wrap. The tummy and the waist have so many fat cells clustered together that it is more difficult for essential oils to penetrate here. A cling-film wrap will aid the penetration of essential oils as well as encourage the elimination of water by causing the skin to sweat.

A cling film wrap can be left in place for one or two hours, but for best results leave overnight, perhaps prior to a special occasion, when you want to squeeze into a figure hugging item of clothing.

Firstly massage the waist, with a blend of essential oils, such as the lemon grass blend or the juniper blend and then wrap a sizeable length of cling-film around the waist and tummy. If left on overnight the essential oils will be unable to evaporate and will be forced into the skin. The skin will also sweat because of the close proximity of the plastic. After use, the cling-film should be cut and discarded. This is not a permanent way to banish fat from the tummy and waist but ideal for- an instant tone-up and is a technique used in many beauty salons.

The Solar Plexus

The solar plexus is sited halfway between the navel and the end of the breastbone, and is a very sensitive area. If we are under stress or have experienced something traumatic (even watching the news on television) we may find that the area of the solar plexus is sore to touch. You may also find that just under the surface of the skin this part of your abdomen feels tight and hard, as though the muscles have become 'knotted up". This is precisely what has happened but tension in the solar plexus can be very easily massaged away.

Solar Plexus (Self Massage)- Solar Plexus is the seat of anxieties, people prone to anxiety should apply a little massage oil containing in 30ml special carrier oil as mentioned above, 6 drops Lavender oil, 3 drops R. Chamomile and 6 drops Geranium oil, to the area between navel and the sternum. Lie on the bed and rest your hand above the solar plexus and just breathe peacefully for a few minutes. Be aware of the tension under your hand. Can you feel tightness? Is the underlying flesh hard to touch?

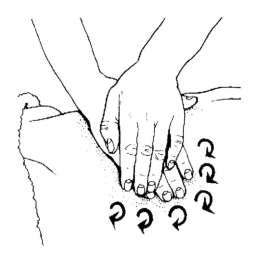

Using both hands, place the fingertips on the solar plexus, so the backs of the fingers are touching each other. Take a deep breath and as you breathe out, gently fingertips to the tender area. As you breathe in, allow the fingers to rise up as the diaphragm expands, and again gently press the fingertips in the solar plexus with the out breath. This is difficult to do if the fingernails are too long.

Continue in this manner for few minutes until the solar plexus has lost its tenderness. Finally apply a little more massage blend and gently rub the abdomen, sweeping your hands in a clockwise circle. Rest for a few minutes, after this or make this solar plexes massage last thing before going to bed, to ensure a restful night.

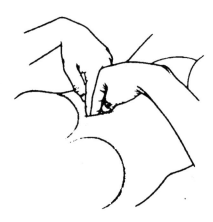

Thighs and Buttocks

The problems: *Thighs, cellulite, fat dull, lifeless skin; excess fat (poor metabolism). Buttocks: Dull lifeless skin, pimples, buttock 'droop'; fat; stretch marks.*

The causes: *Toxins in tissues; lymphatic congestion, stagnation-poor circulation, lack of exercise; poor metabolism, insufficient nutrition-inside and out.*

The solutions: *Aromatic bathing; skin brushing; friction massage moisturizing and nourishing the skin.*

Cellulite

Cellulite is the term used to describe the pitted appearance of the skin when it is pinched between the fingers, "orange peel" is an accurate description of the problem, and in France it is known as 'peau d'orange'. The nickname of 'culotte de cheval' has also been given to the condition, as cellulite is most often found on the outside of the thighs, which can give our legs the appearance of wearing "Jodhpuris". The sense of touch can also detect the presence of cellulite as the skin can be very tender to the touch, and if squeezed, very painful.

Cellulite affects almost 60 per cent of women at some stage of the lives. The good news is that cellulite is a condition which is not permanent and can easily be reversed with aroma oils massage. Even though cellulite rarely responds to dieting and does not always respond to exercise, it does respond, fairly rapidly, to massage with specific essential oils. Cellulite is not a true disease, in the sense of an irreversible pathological change, but a visual warning that the body is not functioning properly (It should not be confused with cellulitis). Less than beautiful buttocks are trying to tell you that the fat cells are accumulating onto buttocks and upper arms. Since, the body sends all of the excess toxins that it cannot manage to eliminate through the lymph, blood stream, liver and kidneys, and normal elimination process, into the extremities of the body, away from the vital

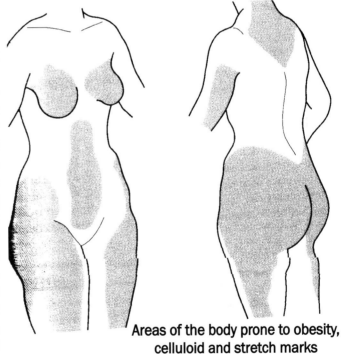

Areas of the body prone to obesity, celluloid and stretch marks

organs. So it seems that buttocks and upper arms are used as a rubbish dump of the body.

Another contributing factor to the development of cellulite is any form of chronic stress, resulting in nervous anxiety. When the body is suffering with severe stress it does not function efficiently, especially when we 'eat for comfort', the excess toxins that the body cannot deal with end up on the thighs and upper arms. The skin is the mirror of internal health, congestion of the skin is often symptomatic of poor circulation, as it is the circulating blood which brings a supply of oxygen that helps elimination of toxins at the fundamental level. This helps cellular regeneration and allows them to functioning healthily.

Essential oils have the ability to decongest tissues and help the body to eliminate toxins, and often works on the internal problems as well as skin conditions. Essential oils of Juniper berry and Lavender are very powerful antiseptic, at the same time act gently on the skin, you can use these for baths and massage. Cellulite is a sign of congestion, visible on the skin, but the organs of elimination are affected. A Lemongrass blend or juniper blend, when used in massage to the affected areas, has a draining effect and stimulates the flow of lymph.

In order to create an optimum situation for eliminating toxins, fats and excess water from the thighs and buttocks, the thighs must be skin brushed thoroughly, taking care also to brush the 'knicker line'- the area of the body where the inguinal nodes are to be found. Stimulation of this area, followed by friction massage with specific essential and fatty oils, is a most effective way to banish cellulite from the thighs.

A suitable recipe is-

5 drops Juniper berry oil
5 drops Rosemary oil
 5 drops Grapefruit oil
5 drops Cypress oil
5 drops Fennel seed oil

Add them to 30 ml of Chosen carrier oil having at least 25% jojoba oil and 10 % Avocado Oil

Obesity

Obesity is the result of eating far more calories than our body can burn up through daily activity, instead of being used as fuel for energy, the fat cells become full rather like a greedy hamster's store cupboard, where the pile of food is never used up, but continues to grow-and the bulkier we become. The saying 'you are what you eat' is unfortunately very true.

Sitting for long periods every day and sedentary work are major factors in loss of muscles tone in the buttocks. Toxins and fats are squashed by the weight of the body pressing down on a relatively small area-the buttocks. The upper thighs also suffer from prolonged periods of sitting, especially the back of the thighs where the circulation can be seriously impaired by pressure from the edge of a chair.

In obesity, lack of muscles tone and fatty deposits respond well to physical massage, especially when used with essential oils that have a stimulating effect on metabolism, such as grapefruit oil for the gall bladder, juniper for the kidneys, lemon orange for the liver. A lemongrass blend or a juniper blend used in regular massage on the thighs and buttocks has a very toning and slimming effect.

You can also try the following oils for a daily massage therapy-

> 5 drops Juniper berry oil
> 5 drops Lemongrass oil
> 5 drops Grapefruit oil
> 5 drops Lemon oil oil
> 5 drops Rosemary oil

Add them to 30 ml of Chosen carrier oil having at least 15% jojoba oil and 10 % Avocado Oil

Stretch marks

If the living skin is considerably overstretched by rapid weight gain or loss, ruptures can occur in the structure of the corium which become visible as pale, silvery stripes, so-called "distension striae", commonly known as 'stretch-marks'. Stretch marks often accompany cellulite or excess fat in the thighs.

The corium is a dense network of collagen fibers, intermingled with elastic fibers which allows the skin to stretch and return to normal. The cells which originate in the basal layer of the epidermis undergo step-by-step transformation, leading to the migration of cells from the basement layer to the surface, a process which takes about 30 days. This means that by applying essential and fatty oils in generous amounts, over a period of time we will be able to influence the new growth of cells which will replace the ruptured skin tissue, and the stretch marks will eventually disappear.

With all problems of the thighs, massage with lemongrass blend or juniper blend can be very successful. Once you've tackled the cellulite and reduced the- excess fat, massage with the following blend-

> 5 drops Cedarwood
> 5 Drops Geranium
> 5 Drops Lavender
> 5 Drops Rosemary
> 5 Drops Vertiver

in 50 Ml. chose base oil addition of 10 % calendula helps the stretch marks to recede and become less visible.

Aromatic Bathing-

The morning is an ideal time of day to tackle cellulite and excess fat of thighs and buttocks. Skin brushing followed by massage with stimulating essential oils, if used late at night, may interfere with your ability to fall asleep, but works better in the morning.

Add to the bath those essential oils which are refreshing and uplifting. The zest of oranges or Mandarin, is a natural choice to revitalize and set the mood for positive action. To this you could add a few drops of Geranium, if your emotions need a 'lift'.

Although some essential oils have specific effects on the body-such as the diuretic properties of juniper oil, it is not necessary to use these oils in the bath, if you are applying liberal quantities of these essential oils in massage. Just choose oils, which will refresh and cleanse the skin in preparation for a massage. Ideal candidates would be Mandarin, Geranium or Rosemary.

Massage of the Thigh-

Take the massage oil of your choice like Juniper Blend, or the one with Lemongrass or Vertiver in blend. Apply the chosen oil, a little at a time, to one thigh, notice how it seeps, into the skin. Beginning just above the knee, work the oil into the skin in small patches, and continue to build up further areas of oiled skin until the entire thigh has been covered. Reposition your leg as necessary, to gain access to every part of the thigh. Using fingertip pressure, stroke the fingers up the leg, not too forcefully and t not too gently also. You will be able to feel areas of discomfort, knobbles of fat under the skin, or crystals of salt etc. Continue to apply more of the massage oil blend, working it into any 'problem areas'. Be sensitive to your body, spending more time massaging sore spots, before sweeping the palm of the hand up the thigh to the top of the leg, and finish up stroking the fingers around the 'knicker line'.- area of inguinal nodes. Apply massage oil to the inguinal and massage for a few minutes, using your finger tips followed by pumping action. This area may feel sensitive and tender to the touch. The preferred blend to use, is the Lemongrass blend, as we want to 'spring clean' the connective tissue and allow the powerful Lemongrass oil to 'burn up' the toxins which have accumulated over the years, the added essences of citrus oils will cleanse, detoxify and help the body's lymphatic system to drain more easily.

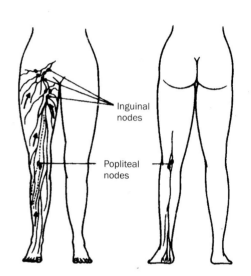

Inguinal nodes

Popliteal nodes

Massage of the buttocks-

If your buttocks have lost their youthful curves, and the cheeks no longer have firm definition but droop and merge ingloriously into the back of the thighs, then this area deserves a lot of attention. It is possible to rejuvenate the buttocks and bring back a firm contour, but only by consistent effort of working on this area with the massage oil blends.

Use either the Lemongrass blend or the Juniper blend with Cypress oil. Massage the oil into one buttock, more oil as it is absorbed by the skin. The best way to self massage the buttocks is to be semi-reclining. Lie on top of your bed, on your side, with buttock to be worked on uppermost, and leg bent.

Use fingertip massage to work the oil blend into the entire skin surface, paying particular attention to the area where buttock meets thigh. Use firm strokes here and work on any portion of skin that feels knotty or lumpy under the surface. Press and probe the flesh in this area, which has been squashed and flattened for so many years of being sat on. After only a few massage sessions focusing on this area, a definite difference can be seen in the shape and definition of the cheeks. If the buttocks are massaged regularly, it is possible to regain a youthful contour to the buttocks.

Knees, Ankles and Feet

The problems- *Fat knees, puffy knees, wrinkly knees. Puffy ankles, hidden ankles, Corns and callous, cracked feet, tired feet, nail bed infections,.*

The causes- *Poor metabolism, hormonal imbalances, excess fat, dehydrated skin, age, ill fitting shoes, neglect.*

The solutions- *Aromatic bathing, skin brushing, massage, foot bath.*

Knees

Even a woman with the most shapely legs and gorgeous figure can feel let down by her knees, especially when her legs are bare. Fortunately the essential oils can work on a deeper level on the skin of the knees, just as they can work on the face or any other part of the body. The most common problems are fat knees, puffy-looking knees, or wrinkly knees. In all knee problems, aromatic bathing and skin brushing are the first step, followed by massage with a well chosen blend of essential and fatty oils.

Aromatic bathing and skin brushing-
The choice of the oils here is not so crucial, so choose one you particularly enjoy. The emphasis is on skin brushing. Take your nail brush and brush up the leg from ankles to knees, using medium pressure. Then brush across and around the knee as well as underneath the knee, where the popliteal lymph nodes lie. Next, bend the knee, and with firmer pressure, brush the top of the knee from all sides, and take the brush strokes about a third of the way up the thigh. Finish the skin brushing by stroking the bristles along the 'knicker line' to inguinal nodes.

The skin may look pink and feel hot, which is a good sign because blood is being brought to the surface of the skin. This has two effects; it brings nutrients to the skin surface and it prepares the skin for the essential oil massage.

Fat knees- Massage with the Lemongrass blend (recipe given in the previous chapter) is excellent for those with fat knees, as it decongests and detoxifies the area. Jojoba may also be used alone since it penetrates quickly and deeply into the skin and it is able to emulsify fats very effectively.

Puffy knees- Massage with the Juniper blend (refer to previous chapter for recipe) is helpful for any one, who experiences fluid retention around the knees. This is a common but easily resolved problem so take heart.

Wrinkly knees- Age and dry skin produce knees that look a little wrinkled. Like wrinkles on the face, a firm massage with the Vertiver oil blend (containing 7 Drops Vertiver, 3 drops Geranium, 3 drops Cedarwood, 3 drops Lavender in 2 tablespoons of chosen base oil) can help restore a youthful, firm texture to these trouble spots.

Massage of the knees- For any knee problem massage the entire knee area with your chosen blend. Using fingertips, feel for any little knots, lumps, toxic deposits or unwanted fat. Massage your knee in small circular movements from underside of the knee, to about a third of the way up to the thigh. With both thumbs placed on the leg above the knee, work outwards and downwards towards the underside of the knees and to the lymph nodes. Continue for up to 10 minutes on each knee.

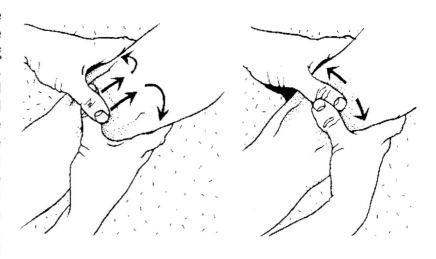

Ankles and feet

Being further away, from the torso than the knees, the ankles and feet can easily accumulate fluids (especially pre-menstrual), fats and toxins. Dry brushing and foot soak with essential oils, followed by scrubbing and massage with aroma oils is very helpful.

Foot Baths and Skin Brushing- You can use any essential oils blend for foot bath. In the summer time, Peppermint with Rosemary is very cooling and uplifting combination, In the winter oils of Myrtle with Black pepper are comforting and warming. Anyone who suffers from foot odor could use Cypress, Juniper or Frankincense, since these oils have natural deodorant properties.

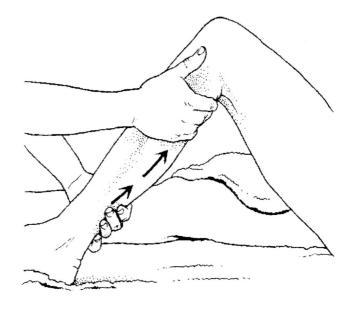

With a nail brush, brush the top of the foot from the toes to the ankle, paying particular attention to the area around the inside and outside of the ankle bone. Most of the lymph from the foot drains to the popliteal nodes, but some lymph vessels go directly to the inguinal nodes. Therefore, stimulate both areas with the nail brush.

Puffy ankles

Make a foot soak containing 3 drops each of Juniper berry, Cypress and Pine needle oil, follow it with gentle massage. Juniper blend is wonderfully effective as juniper is a good diuretic and helps drain fluid from this area. Long hours of standing or after a party or other occasion when larger than normal quantities of alcohol have been consumed, the ankles become a little puffy- this is the body's way of saying it is having difficulty in coping with the alcohol. Drinking extra glasses of water is a valuable aid to your body's elimination system, as is a massage with diuretic essential oil blend.

Hidden ankles

Excess fat or water retention is the cause of hidden ankles. You can either massage with the Lemongrass blend or Juniper blend to help uncover ankle bones you had forgotten you had.

Massage of the ankles and feet- Apply the chosen oils to the top and sides of one foot and ankle. With firm fingertip pressure, stroke from the toes to the ankle, and then draw your fingers around the ankle. Continue these movements for several minutes. Apply the maximum pressure, you find is bearable; some of us have very sensitive feet and ankles, but the massage should have a degree of firmness. If the feet and ankles are massaged on a regular basis, they do become less tender to the touch as toxins and fluids are removed. Finish the massage by smoothing the skin up to the knees, so that the lymph is encouraged to drain. As some lymph vessels drain directly into the inguinal nodes, be sure to massage this area as well. Many women experience swelling and tenderness of the flesh just below the ankle bone immediately prior to menstruation, and gentle massage of this area will help the body to release tissue fluids.

Tired feet

Lots of tension is stored in the feet, not to mention the trauma of teetering around on high heels, or simply standing on and using your relatively tiny feet. They need a treat from time to time. Nothing is lovelier than an aromatic foot soak. Place your feet in a few inches of warm water in the bottom of your bath tub or in a separate bowl to which a few drops of essential oil have been added- lavender, geranium, ylang-ylang, rose, bergamot, the choice is yours.

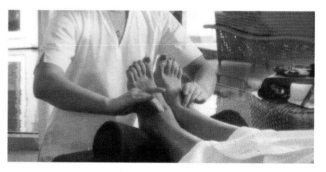

After a 10 minutes soak, use a pumice stone to smooth away dry skin from the heels and toes. Cover one knee- with a towel and put your other foot up for a massage. Clench your fist and, starting at the base of the toes, draw your knuckles along the length of the foot to the heel. Cover the whole foot with knuckle caresses, which stimulate many foot reflex points and release tension. Change towel to opposite knee and your other foot. Dry feet with a towel and apply a little jojoba oil. You should feel as though you are walking on air.

Corns and callous

Corn and callous are result of the ill fitting foot wear causing friction at the pressure zones at the sole of the foot resulting into hardening of skin. Direct application of Tea Tree or in combination with Oregano and Calendula is quite useful. You can also use Salicylic acid (or aspirin powder) make a paste and apply at the corn or use corn plaster on which keep dripping a drop or two of tea tree oil.

Cracked feet

Pressure of the body weight, excessive dryness and metabolic deficiency causes the cracking of the skin especially around heals. Soaking, moisturizing and nourishing feet, is helpful in correcting this condition. Beeswax, jojoba oil, Almond oil, water and essential oils are useful ingredients to make an emollient and protective foot cream.

Take 15gms Beeswax (finely chopped)
add 1 Tablespoon Jojoba oil
and 3 tablespoons of Almond oil
place in a bowl on double burner at medium heat, allowing to melt, stir occasionally.

After it has melted remove the bowl. Let it cool a bit add a little hot water (at the same temperature) whisk to make an emulsion, add essential oils and store in a jar keep at a cool place away from light and heat.

Alternatively use 1 Teaspoon Almond oil, 1 Tea spoon Jojoba and 1 Teaspoon Avocado oil as base to which you can add- 3 drops Vertiver, 3 drops patchouli, 3 drops Lavender. Apply thoroughly after a foot soak.

Nail Bed Infections

Mostly nail bed infections are fungal in nature, either due to wearing synthetic socks or moisture. Best treatment is to use neat Tea tree oil, apply on nail 1-2 drops two to three times daily. You can also use Tea tree oil in foot soak, follow with foot massage, then apply additional Tea tree oil on the affected nails.

ATHLETE'S FOOT AND RINGWORM

These are both contagious fungal infections characterized by red, flaky skin and itching. Athlete's foot occurs between the toes, sometimes affecting the toenails. Ringworm, which forms a circle on the skin, generally affects the scalp, knees, elbows or between the fingers. Let the skin breathe by avoiding tight clothes and nylon socks.

*Make a blend using 1 teaspoon almond oil, 1drop each of Lavender, Oregano, Myrrh and Tea tree and apply at least 3 times a day. Tea tree may also be applied neat (or diluted in a gel) - check sensitization first by patch test.

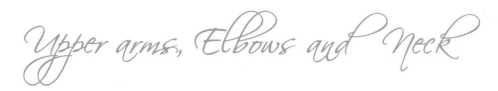

Upper arms, Elbows and Neck

The Problems- *Flabby upper arms, cellulite, obesity, wrinkled elbows, rough or dead skin on elbows, dehydrated skin, stored up tension in neck, lines on neck.*

The causes- *Loss of muscle tone, toxins, poor metabolism, age, pressure of leaning (elbows), emotional, mental stress and poor circulation.*

The solutions- *Bathing, skin brushing, massage, astringent mask, moisturizing.*

Aromatic baths- Bathing in aromatic water is beneficial for all problems relating to the upper arms, elbows and neck. Only a few drops of essential oil to a full tub of water are needed to create a therapeutic bath which will cleanse the skin, relax tense muscles, and open up the pores of the skin in readiness to receive massage oils. *Many essential oils are excellent for the skin but especially recommended for their therapeutic properties and their fragrance are Rosemary, Orange, Myrtle, Juniper berry Ginger and Lavender.*

Skin brushing- releases toxins from the body by the gentle stimulation of the skin's surface, and when incorporated into the aromatic bathing ritual, transforms the process of taking a bath into an important health and beauty treatment.

Take a nail brush, and brush from wrist to elbow, gently at first, as many times as it takes to cover the entire forearm. Then repeat using firmer pressure. Gently brush the folds of the elbow, where the cubital nodes are housed. These lymph glands are the first line of defense in detoxifying our hands, nails and forearms, and can become swollen and painful if we have a problem such as a septic, swollen and painful fingers. Now sweep from the bend of the elbow up to the top of the arm, if necessary lifting up your arm so that you can brush the underside. Continue the gentle brushing and sweeping the armpit, so that the auxiliary nodes are encouraged to work efficiently in carrying away the waste material dislodged by massage. Finally, sweep across the top of your shoulder, from the base round to finish where the arm meets the body, relax in the aromatic water for five minutes or so. Repeat, on the other arm.

The neck can also be skin brushed in the bath, with the brush stroking downwards from under the skin of the chin to the base of the neck. Work your way around the neck until all the skin, even the back of the neck, has been brushed. Next, sweep the brush from the back of the neck round to the front, finishing where the two ends of the clavicle meet. Using slightly firmer strokes, brush from the shoulder across front of the chest, under the clavicle, and end at the top of the sternum. Repeat on the other side of the body.

Cellulite on upper arms

Cellulite on the upper arms is your body's 'overflow' tip where it has dumped toxins that it cannot deal with in other ways. *Essential oils blends of Lemongrass or Juniper, (refer to chapter on Thighs & buttocks) will remove toxins from the connective tissues, deep cleanse and disinfect the dermis and bring a fresh supply of blood to the surface of skin, helping the circulatory system to carry away unwanted debris.*

Excess fat on upper arms

Too much fat on the upper arms probably occurs in tandem with too much fat on other parts of the body. *The Lemongrass blend is most suitable for massage,* in this case. Allow your fingertips to detect the condition of the underlying skin, feel the lumps under the surface and encourage them to go away. If there are tiny spots or hard crystal like deposits under the skin, encourage their removal and elimination by massage.

Flabby upper arms

We say that something is 'flabby' when it has lost its tone and has succumbed to the forces of gravity. Flabby upper arms are usually to be seen on women who have lost not only weight but also muscles tone, either from age or from crash dieting, allowing the skin to hang in folds. *Some improvement in the appearance of the upper arms can be achieved with massage of the skin with lemongrass blend combined with few drops of Cypress oil.* However, it will only be possible to effect a very gradual change in the condition and appearance of the skin, and best results will be achieved if a little light exercise is also incorporated.

Dry Skin

Dry, wrinkly skin is the easiest of the upper arm problems to rectify, as dry skin denotes a lack of oils in the skin. Skin cells are constantly renewing themselves, as the old, dead cells are removed from the surface of our bodies; new cells are already being pushed upwards, towards the surface. By feeding the skin with pure oils, both essential and fatty, we can feed the deeper layers where the cells are formed, giving them the ideal conditions for birth and growth. *Essential oils of Vertiver, Sandalwood, Cedar wood combined with base oils of Almond, Wheat germ and jojoba oil, will give the skin all the nourishment it requires, whilst the Vertiver in the blend will encourage the cells to absorb and retain moisture, making and more youthful.*

Massage of upper arms-

Whether your upper arm problem is cellulite, excess fat, flabby loose skin, or rough dry skin, the massage technique is the same. Massage of the upper arms, following an aromatic bath and skin brushing, is the most effective way to get essential oils into skin.

With your choice of massage blend, apply the oil to the upper left arm, from the elbow to the shoulder, covering all of the skin, underarm included. Rest the left wrist and hand across the top of the head-this will enable you to massage the underarm more easily. Using only your fingertips, smooth and stroke the skin from the elbow to the armpit, with short and repetitive strokes, like sweeping leaves along the ground. Be sensitive to your body and feel for any little fatty bumps, crystals or pimples under the surface, and massage these areas thoroughly. Apply more oil blend whenever necessary. Dropping your arm down by your side, massage the outer edge of your, arm from elbow to shoulder, smoothing away the lumps and bumps.

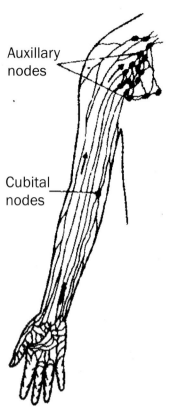

Now turn the arm so that the palm is facing upwards and massage the biceps. Again, using fingertip massage, work the oil blend into the skin from elbow to shoulder. Finish by massaging the entire armpit area, and help your auxiliary glands to carry out their important function.

Do not shave, wax or use depilatory cream on the underarms immediately before or after massage of upper arms and underarm area.

Elbows

It is often said that a person's true age can be determined by looking at her elbow, because the elbows cannot be cosmetically enhanced and cared for in the way that the face can.

The flesh covering the elbow is, by necessity, fairly loose fitting, as elbows have to bend. It can therefore easily lose elasticity and become wrinkled. Whatever problem we experience with the condition of our elbows and upper arms, a regular ,massage with chosen essential oil blend, in the morning and night, will definitely help, it may take some time to have a noticeable improvement both in appearance and the feel of the elbows.

Puffy fat elbows
Puffy and fat elbows are unlikely to be found in isolation, and will be part of an overall excess of adipose tissue in the body. The true solution for puffiness lies in eating healthily and increasing the body's metabolism, but a useful aromatic adjunct is to massage the elbows with the Juniper blend of oils in combination with the citrus oils of Grapefruit and Orange oils, which are cleansing and stimulating to the tissues, helping the lymph to take away fluids and proteins and return them to the circulatory system where they may be further broken down and eliminated from the body. For excess fat in elbow area it is better to use Lemon grass blend.

Hard, dry and wrinkled elbows
As with dry upper arms, the problem of dry elbows is a lack of natural oil, which in mature skins is added by a breakdown in connective tissue and inability to retain moisture. The blend of Vertiver in jojoba is a wonderful combination for massaging dry, wrinkled elbows, since Vertiver can help the skin cells to attract and hold water more easily. Sandalwood is another very useful oil for massaging into dry skin, or try cleansing the elbows with a cotton wool pad soaked in sandalwood aromatic water and then massage in a little of the Vertiver blend.

Massage of elbows-

The main problems with the elbows are puffy or fat elbows and hard, dry and wrinkled skin. Although seemingly different, the cause is fairly constant buildup of toxins, fluids or fats due to inadequate lymph drainage and lack of physical care. Massage of the elbows and stimulation of the cubital lymph nodes (in the fold of the elbow) will help to bring about a more healthful, youthful appearance. Whatever the individual problem, the massage technique is the same. Fingertip massages, using the chosen aromatic blend and lots of it - is required in the area of the elbow.

Pour a little blended oil into a small massage bowl. Sit on the edge of your bed or chair with the left arm crossing in front of your body and the left hand resting of your right hand and smooth into the skin around the elbow. Using fingertips, massage the flesh around the bony part of the elbow, feeling how much or how little flesh is covering the bone. Whilst smoothing in the oil, feel for any little bumps or hard spots under the surface of the skin. These are not supposed to be there and denote the presence of pockets of toxins, excess proteins, knotted fibers and crystal deposits. Now, with your fingertips, stroke and rub the skin on and around the elbow, giving extra attention to rough or lumpy areas. Continue the fingertip massage for about 15 minutes, or until your right hand feels tired. Then, stretching out your knees, massage the inner elbow where, the cubital lymph nodes are housed. These nodes are responsible for the health of our forearms, hands and nails, filtering away poisons and producing lymphocytes. Using the flat of your hand stroke the flesh upwards from below the elbow to the top of the arm and finally spend a minute or so massaging the nodes at the top of the arm be lifting up the left arm and rubbing the nodes at the junction of the arm and the torso. Now change hands and massage the right arm in the same way.

Neck

Whether long and sleek or short and thick, our neck supports our head, enables us to see around corners, and is a place of adornment. Like the elbows, the flesh covering the neck has to be fairly loose in order that we may have 180 degree flexibility to the left and right. The skin of the neck is a dense network of collagen fibers, intermingled with elastic fibers, which enable the skin to stretch and, then return to normal. Small enough to be encircled by our two hands, the neck houses an incredible collection of bones, veins arteries, nerves, glands, lymph nodes and ducts, as well as the gullet and windpipe. The muscles of the neck have to support the weight of the head (around 4 kg) which is why too much strain or tension in the neck produces a headache. Emotional or mental stress aggravate the condition.

Stretching the neck from time to time is beneficial to the muscles and the blood flow, and is especially important if our job causes us to sit for many hours a day with our heads facing in one direction, such as in front of Computer or TV screen. Massaging the neck is also important for several reasons; to release tension from the muscles; to encourage the free flow of lymph, and the efficient drainage of waste products from the head, face and the neck itself; to allow good blood circulation; and to prevent any impingement of nerves. Looking after the neck is much more than just a cosmetic routine to enhance our physical beauty-it is a sensible way to keep the face, the head and the whole of the body in a good state of health.

Lines and loose skin

The neck should ideally be cleansed and moisturized every night as part of the daily care plan for the face. The skin on the neck, like the skin of the face, is subject to contact with polluted air and the elements, and will need to be thoroughly cleansed every day. After cleansing, apply 3 drops Vertiver, 3 drops Lavender, 3 drops Rosemary in 1 tablespoon of Olive and jojoba blend, using large, firm sweeps, massage into the sides of the neck . With long hair pinned up, massage the back of the neck, at the occipital area, from the hairline down to the shoulders, and rub away at any sore spots your fingers may discover. There are many lymph nodes in the neck which draw of toxins from the face and head.

Neck Massage

Ideally the front of the neck should be cleansed and massaged everyday at the same time as your face. In this way the skin stands the very best chance of retaining its elasticity and staying free from lines. However, the back of the neck will only need to be massaged periodically, such as when you have a headache, or when you want your neck and shoulders to look as good as your face.

By massaging the back of the neck with a massage oil blend, we can release a lot of tension, relax sore and tight muscles, and encourage the dispersion of toxins and static energy, so easily accumulated by hours of desk work, driving, worrying over problems, or even just by sleeping in the wrong position at night.

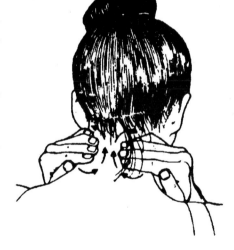

You can even use neat Lavender oil for the purpose, as Lavender releases the stiffness of the muscles. Alternatively prepare a blend using essential oils of Lavender, Myrtle, Rosemary, Juniper berry and Geranium in base oil of Olive, Grape seed and Avocado.

Apply a little of this blend, to the fingertips and place your hands on the back of your neck so that your fingers meet on the vertebral column. Now draw the fingers down, round and up so that the neck is being covered in large circles, and continue to do this for as long as you feel comfortable. Next, stretch hands even further down the back of the neck and starting at the spine and applying firm pressure, down your fingers round the bottom of your neck until they reach the right angle between neck and shoulder.

Repeat this move several times as it is a very effective way of removing tension and allows energy to flow to the head. Next, place fingertips at base of neck and slide them up the back of the neck, with fingers on either side of the spine. When your fingers reach the hairline, apply stronger pressure and hold for a count of five. Allow your fingers to press and soothe all sore spots along the occipital (where the skull joins the neck) and continue outwards until your hands reach your ears. Then, taking the back of the neck between fingers and thumb, squeeze gently, allowing your fingers and thumb, to slide across the skin and meet at the spinal column. Finish the massage by stroking the fingers from the top to the bottom of the neck and applying firm pressure to the lymph nodes below the clavicle.

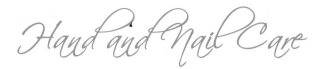

Hand and Nail Care

The problems- Dry skin, dehydrated skin, fat or puffy hands, brittle nails, ridged nails.

The causes- Lack of moisture, insufficient sebum production, environment, diet.

The solution- Aromatic hand bath, nail soaks, moisturizing, massage barrier cream.

Hands

Hands and face are the two areas of our body most often exposed to the elements, while we protect our facial skin with moisturizers and make-up, our hands are often neglected and become damaged. There is only a thin layer of flesh over the bones of the hand; the back of our hands can age more quickly than the skin of the face. Even if we are blessed with a youthful-looking face, our hands can instantly reveal our true age.

There are two ways to improve your hands.
1. A barrier cream that can be applied regularly throughout the day.
2. Nightly moisturizing routine with rejuvenating oils and aromatic waters.

Daytime barrier cream

A barrier cream has two functions. One is to provide an invisible film or barrier against the environment- the weather, central heating or AC and water in all its usages (washing up, washing our hair, handling the laundry), etc. The second is to soften and moisturize dry skin and to feed it with nourishing fatty oils and essential oils.

Beeswax, jojoba oil, Almond oil, water and essential oils are the ingredients necessary to make an emollient and protective hand cream which is not very expensive.

Take 15gms Beeswax (finely chopped)
add 1 Tablespoon Jojoba oil
and 3 tablespoons of Almond oil
place in a bowl on double burner at medium heat, allowing to melt, stir occasionally.

After it has melted remove the bowl. Let it cool a bit add a little hot water (at the same temperature) whisk to make an emulsion, add essential oils and store in a jar keep at a cool place away from light and heat.

Being simple to make, and not containing any preservatives, it is preferable to make a batch every three to four weeks, rather than make a large quantity.

There is a huge range of essential oils, which could be chosen for their fragrance, as well as their ability to soften and protect the skin, for example Vertiver and Lavender or Geranium with sandalwood. Warm, earthy aromas make a pleasing bouquet when blended, such as Vertiver, Patchouli and Sandalwood.

Night time rejuvenating hand massage

Massage the hands before going to bed using Vertiver oil blend. Hold your left hand with your right, and with the right thumb massage the back of the hand using small circular movements, working between the carpel bones. Take one finger of your left hand between the fingers and thumb of your right hand and massage the entire length of the finger. Rub your palms together and smooth the oil into the entire hand and wrist. Repeat on other hand. Next, pour a little sandalwood aromatic water or Rose Water into the palm of one hand. Carefully rub the aromatic water into both hands, as if you were washing your hands. When dry, apply a little more Vertiver oil blend. After massaging the hands, spend a few minutes massaging the lymph nodes situated in the elbow area.

Hand bath

Hands that are dry, rough or damaged can be healed and softened by the use of an aromatic hand bath. Any of the essential oils which are beneficial for dry skin may be used, such as Sandalwood, Rose, Vertiver, Lavender, Geranium, or patchouli. Alternatively use a combination of Rose water with little Glycerine.

To prepare a hand bath, you will need a bowl that is large enough to place your hands in for half an hour; a casserole dish may prove to be the correct size. Essential oils differ in their ability to disperse in water and if using one of the viscous oils- Sandalwood, Vertiver or Patchouli- it will first be necessary to mix them with a thinner oil such as Lavender, Geranium or Palmarosa. Place essential oils in the bowl, add warm water and allow your hands to soak for 10-15 minutes.

Choose any of the following combinations -1 drop Vertiver
      1 drop Sandalwood
      2 drops Geranium
      Or
      2 drops Rose
      2 drops Lavender
      2 drops Bergamot

Pat hands dry with a clean towel and apply a liberal amount of jojoba oil. Massage into the hands, as if washing your hands with the oil, until your hands have absorbed as much jojoba as possible. Rub excess oil onto any other area of dry skin such as the elbows or knees, or alternatively blot the excess with a tissue.

The Nails

The nail is composed of keratin, as is the skin; it is a horny plate of the epidermis. It consists of cornified scales, overlapping like roof tiles. The nail bed is the living part of the nail and consists of connective tissue channels that carry blood vessels along the nail's length, from the half moon to the fingertip. It is the flow of blood beneath the surface of the nail which gives the pink or red tinge. The nail projecting from the finger tip is completely dead, which enables us to cut and file our nails without experiencing pain.

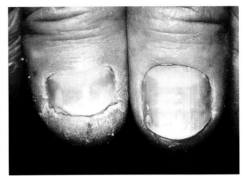

Nothing much can be done to increase the strength of the nail once it has grown beyond the fingertip, but much can be done to grow healthy nails in the nail bed. When nails are dry and brittle and split easily, it is simply because they are not receiving sufficient 'food' in order for them to grow. Vitamin A supplement also help to improve the condition of nails. The aromatic way to bring nutrients to the nail bed is to use a hypereamic oil, such as Myrtle, either in the form of a massage oil or as a nail soak.

Massage oil for nails

A simple but effective, massage oil for nails can be prepared in minutes as under -

> 1 Tablespoon Sweet Almond Oil
> 1 Teaspoon Wheat germ Oil
> 1 Teaspoon Jojoba Oil
> 4 drops Lavender Oil
> 3 drops Geranium Oil
> 2 drops Sandalwood Oil.

Dip the fingertips into the mixture so that some oil goes under the nail. Next, massage the oil into the nail wall, half moon and up to the first joint of the finger. When mixture has begun to be absorbed, put your fingertips together so that your hands form a sphere, and gently press the nails of the right hand underneath the nails of the left hand. Hold for a few seconds. Then press the nails of the left hand under the nails of the right hand.

Aromatic nail soak

An alternative to using the massage oil for the nails is to soak the fingertips in a pot of warm water containing -

> 2 drops Lavender oil
> 2 drops Niaouli oil
> 3 drops Wheat Germ or Vitamin E oil (optional).

Both Lavender and Niaouli are tissue stimulants, and promote the growth of new skin- one of the reasons why they are used to heal burns. By soaking the fingertips in this aromatic liquid (especially if Vitamin E is included), a highly nutritious meal is provided for our nails. Allow nails to soak for 10-20 minutes, depending on how starved your nails are. Rinse your hands in clear water after soaking, pat dry, and massage in a little jojoba oil or aromatic barrier cream.

Section IV
TREATMENTS OF COMMON AILMENTS

First Aid & Muscular Problems

Infections & Respiratory Illnesses

Stress Related Conditions

Women's Health

Babies, Infants & Children

Beauty (Skin, Skin conditions & Hair Care) & Pleasure

Treatments of Common Ailments

Aromatherapy is the art and science of healing and rejuvenation. It is much more than bath or shower gels, it can be used by all therapists medical /non medical, as a complementary therapy for prevention and treatment of all common and chronic ailments. As mentioned in earlier chapters aromatherapy oils and products boost the immune level, help eliminate toxins at fundamental level, also help the healing besides providing specific therapeutic effect as per the property of the oil used.

Following common conditions respond very well to Aromatherapy oils.-

First Aid-Cuts, burns, bumps, insect bites, sprains, cramps etc.

Beauty Care- Facial Care delays aging wrinkling, under eye dark circles, pigmentation and scars/marks. In Hair Care- Controls dandruff, falling and graying of Hair.

Chakra Healing/ Balancing- Essential oils are the subtle life force of the plant and present most appropriate and potent tool for Chakra healing and balancing.

INFECTIONS- Essential oils are reputed to be anti infectious, anti-bacterial, anti-viral, anti-fungal therefore very effective in post operative care.

Skin Disorders- Eczema, Psoriasis, <u>Fungal Infections, Unhealing Ulcers, Bed Sores</u>, Boils, Acne, herpes, corns, warts, Scars, Sunburns, Nail bed infections etc.

Muscular Problems- Aches, Pains, Sprains, cramps, Rheumatism, Arthritis and Bursitis (tennis elbow) etc.

Circulatory Problems- Blood Pressure related (High / Low), Palpitation, Hyper Tension, Varicose Veins, Piles/Fistula etc.

Respiratory Conditions- Asthma, Bronchitis, Sinusitis, common cold, Respiratory Tract or lung infections etc.

Psychosomatic Conditions- Stress, Anxiety, depression, hypertension, headaches, migraines, Insomnia & Fatigue.

Gynocological Conditions-Candida(Thrush) Leucorrhea, cystitis, Pruritis, Oedema, PMS & menstrual (Periods Related) Problems.

Other problems Like Mouth ulcers, tooth & gums infections, Laryngitis, Pharingitis and even digestive problems.

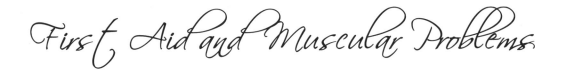

First Aid and Muscular Problems

BRUISES AND BUMPS

LAVENDER oil is one of the best for all bumps, bruises, cramps, sprains. For quick pain relief, and to stop the swelling, apply neat Lavender.

*Minor bruises and bumps can be treated using a cold compress (such as a wet flannel or lint wrapped round an ice cube) to which has been added 3 drops of either lavender, marjoram or geranium.

*If there is inflammation, 2 drops of German chamomile should be applied, along with Lavender, in 1 teaspoon of non-greasy cream or gel.

BURNS (MINOR) AND SUNBURN

*For minor household burns or scalds apply ice-cold water immediately for 10 minutes, then a couple of drops of neat lavender. Renew 3 times daily.

*Large areas of redness from sunburn can be soothed by adding 5-10 drops of German chamomile to a lukewarm bath and soaking for 10 minutes. More severe patches or blisters should be treated with a few drops of neat lavender oil.

*A good after sun treatment, for dry, parched or red skin is to blend 2 drops each of Lavender, Geranium and German Chamomile with 1 tablespoon almond oil or Aloe Gel, massage in well after sunbathing.

CUTS, SORES AND SCARS

Essential oils are very useful for minor first aid since they can reduce the possibility of infection, encourage the skin to heal and help prevent scarring.

*Always clean a cut or sore carefully with a little cooled boiled water to which has been added 2 drops of any of the following antiseptic oils: Lavender, Tea tree, Juniper or Geranium.

*For small cuts or grazes, apply 1-2 drops of neat Lavender as needed. For larger injuries, add a few drops of Lavender to plaster or gauze to cover the wound. Renew the dressing 3 times daily.

For infected cuts or splinters, apply 3 drops of Tea tree or German chamomile diluted in 1 teaspoon of gel to the affected area 3 times daily, especially if there is inflammation.

* If the wound is bleeding, dab it with a gauze, soaked in a bowl of cold water to which has been added 2 drops each of Lavender, Tea Tree & Lemon.

*If the cut or sore is weepy, a drop of the oil of Myrrh, Benzoin or Patchouli may be applied, in combination with Lavender and Tea tree, to the dressing or used to bathe the wound, diluted in warm water.

* For bed sores and unhealing ulcers a combination of Lavender, Tea Tree and German Chamomile with Calendula is very effective.

*If a scar is slow to heal, make an ointment using 3 drops in total of either German chamomile, Lavender or Frankincense (or a combination of these) in 1 teaspoon of wheat germ oil mixed with a little Calendula or Rosehip oil. This should be applied regularly until the skin is healthy again.

INSECT BITES AND REPELLANTS

*To keep insects out of the house, vaporize a combination, of any three of the following oils- Citronella, Lemongrass, Thyme, Peppermint, Lavender, Basil, Eucalyptus, Geranium or Atlas Cedar wood, you can also use them in plant sprays or apply to hanging ribbons.

* An excellent blend can also be made by mixing 2 drops each of Thyme, Lavender and Peppermint with 8 drops of Lemongrass. This can be used as an airborne deterrent blend in an oil burner, vaporizer or plant sprayer, you can also add 6 drops to 1 tablespoon of carrier oil or cream, to be applied, directly to the skin.

*A simple method of keeping insects at bay, especially mosquitoes, is to rub a few drops of neat Lavender on to exposed areas of the skin or on to clothing (it does not stain).

*Oils which keep moths away from linen include Lavender, Patchouli, Camphor, Atlas Cedar wood and basil.

*When it comes to treating bites or stings, the most effective and simple remedy is neat Lavender, applied immediately to the sting and then re-applied at least 3 times a day. This works for mosquitoes, gnats, bees, wasps and ties (as well as nettle rash). For ties, first apply a drop of neat Tea tree to make them lose their grip, before removing.

*If there is a rash, swelling or inflammation, 1 drop of German chamomile and 2 drops of Lavender should be added in 1 teaspoon of non-greasy cream or gel and applied.

MUSCULAR ACHES, PAINS AND SPRAINS

*Muscular pain as a result of over-exertion responds well to local massage. To ease aches and pains use 3 drops each of Lavender, Rosemary, wintergreen and Eucalyptus in 1 tablespoon olive oil, then rub well into the affected areas.

*Soaking in a hot bath is an easy and effective way of bringing instant relief. To aid relaxation and ease pain, add 5-10 drops of Lavender, Eucalyptus Marjoram, Clary sage and German chamomile to the water. Adding Epsom salt to the water, will help to relax the tired muscles.

*To relieve muscle spasm, apply neat Lavender as a first aid or in combination with Marjoram and Eucalyptus in olive oil. Alternatively, add these oils to a hot compress.

*To help prepare the muscles for action and increase muscle tone use 3 drops each of Rosemary and Juniper with 2 drops of Black pepper in 1 tablespoon carrier oil for local massage; or add 5-10 drops of Rosemary, Grapefruit or Juniper to the bath.

*To treat a sprain apply Lavender oil directly or prepare a cold compress to which has been added a few drops of either Lavender or German chamomile (or both), apply to the injury and repeat as often as possible to reduce the swelling. Do not massage. Wrap in a bandage and rest the joint as much as possible.

Pain, Relief with essential oils

Pain often refers to an acute and unpleasant sensation arising from bodily injury or disease. Concepts of pain and pain mechanisms are highly controversial and for that reason all classifications of pain remain quite arbitrary. The bony frame work of the skeleton is covered by voluntary muscles that we can contract or relax at will. In contrast, the involuntary muscles of the heart and digestive system are outside our immediate control. Pain may be experienced either in voluntary or involuntary muscles, however for treatment of any pain the *following three things should be ascertained first-*

- *POISTION of the pain- as accurately as possible, especially the area of greatest severity is often suggestive of the disease.*

- *CHARACTER OR SEVERITY of pain- by finding how it interferes with sleep, pleasure or work.*

- *NATURE of pain- translating as far as possible symptoms into scientific terms. Because diseases which cause little pain in the beginning often end fatally.*

For practical purposes there are two principal types of pain- SUPERFICIAL and DEEP. Pain is sharply localized in superficial structures like muscles and joints or diffusively or poorly localized in deeper structures like heart, digestive system etc. Usually the relief from pain is achieved by removal of the stimulus or neutralization of the effects of the stimulus, and when these are not feasible by dulling or obliterating the sensation of pain.

ESSENTIAL OILS administered for pain relief, work on the muscular system, by neutralizing or removing the stimulus, besides helping to remove the underlying cause of the pain. If the cause of the pain is some disease or illness, in that case only proper diagnosis and treatment can help. Pain also forces the patient to rest the part which is diseased. Nothing can undermine the importance of rest. Indeed REST is the first principle in the treatment of all diseases. Essential oils may be used in addition to relax muscles, relieve pain and cleanse and detoxify the system. Since essential oils work on our body at the fundamental level by- IMPROVING CIRCULATION, INCREASING BODY'S REGENERATION RATE, BY ELIMINATING TOXINS AT FUNDAMENTAL LEVEL. All the essential oils, by nature, are antiseptic, antibacterial, antiviral, disinfectant besides some have special therapeutic properties like anti-inflammatory, warming, stimulating, diuretic, analgesic, muscle relaxant etc. One of the most renowned oil for all kind of pains especially rheumatic pain is the essential oil of Wintergreen mostly used as methyl salicylate (active ingredient of the oil) in all pain balms and liniments. However when we use a combination of aromatherapy oils such as Wintergreen, Eucalyptus, Rosemary, Marjoram, Clove, Lavender, Thyme etc. in a suitable carrier oil, the results are much more efficient.

CRAMPS :-

Temporary muscular spasms during or after physical exertion are not uncommon , but a more long term problem is the type of cramp that occurs in the evening or at night affecting mainly the calf muscles and feet; thought to be due to poor circulation or possibly due to calcium and potassium deficiency. Application of neat Lavender helps in this condition to relieve pain, other useful oils to relieve this type of cramp are- Sweet Marjoram, Basil, Cajuput, Eucalyptus, Rosemary and Chamomile. The essential oils can be mixed, in a suitable base oil and rubbed well in the area. Those who are prone to this type of muscular cramps can make and keep this mix ready and handy, as a preventive measure the oil blend can be applied every night initially, later the frequency can be reduced to every second night then to twice a week; in case cramps return, increase the frequency of application.

SPRAINS :-

 A sprain may occur when ligaments are torn or stretched by a sudden jerky movement. The affected joint becomes swollen and painful. Sprains respond well to aromatherapy treatments, you can use neat Lavender on affected area as a first aid, you should also seek medical attention if there is a doubt of broken or splintered bone. To treat a sprain, prepare a cold compress to which essential oils of Sweet Marjoram, Rosemary, Lavender and German Chamomile are added, apply to the affected area; you can also prepare a mix of these oils in suitable base oil for gentle application of the affected part. Never massage sprained joint. Repeat compress as often as possible to reduce swelling. Wrap in a bandage and rest the affected part as much as possible.

RHEUMATISM, ARTHRITIS AND BURSITIS :-

Rheumatism is a general word for pain and inflammation affecting the joints and surrounding muscles and includes arthritis and bursitis. Arthritis is a term used to describe inflammation of the joints, specifically; there are two main types   RHEUMATOID ARTHRITIS is a chronic inflammation of the connective tissue around joints which causes pain, swelling and stiffness and is often accompanied by weight loss and tiredness. It seems to affect women more than men and unlike osteo arthritis, usually attacks pairs of joints. Conflict on an inner or emotional level often contributes to the development of this disease, as does a poor diet which can lead to a build up, of toxins in the body, with uric acid being deposited as crystals in the joint spaces. Climate is also an important consideration, and the dampness aggravates the condition.

 In severe cases the joints can become crippled and deformed. OSTEO ARTHRITIS is a progressive wearing away of the cartilage which results in severe pain and reduced mobility. The connective tissue thickens and fluid may fill the joint, causing swelling. Aromatherapy can help to relax muscles and relieve pain, but it cannot renew worn cartilage though it can always help to relieve pain. One effective treatment include Evening primrose oil taken 1 teaspoonful (5 ml.) taken orally everyday along with Calcium supplements. Evening primrose not only helps Calcium absorption but also regulates body's physiology.

Bursitis is one of the most common rheumatic conditions, usually affecting the shoulders, elbows (tennis elbow) and knees (housemaid knees). In most cases, the same oils help this condition also.

One of the renowned essential oils for rheumatic conditions is oil of WINTER GREEN, which can be used in conjunction with other oils like German Chamomile. In case of inflammation, Juniper Berry, Eucalyptus, Rosemary, Eucalyptus and Cypress are useful also help to reduce swelling mainly due to edema. The warming properties of Black Pepper, Sweet Marjoram and Ginger help to relax muscles and relieve mild pain.

You can prepare a calming, ant-inflammatory and detoxifying massage oil mix using 5 drops each of Juniper berry, Eucalyptus, Lavender, Pine needles and German Chamomile oil. This mix can be applied with gentle pressure, avoid massage of painful or inflamed joints. Warm baths can also help to relax muscles and relieve pain; just sprinkle a couple of drops of Lavender, Rosemary and Eucalyptus in the bath water. In a hot compress, using a couple of drops of black pepper, Lavender, or Marjoram or a combination of these, helps to ease local pain.

You can prepare a good anti-rheumatic oil, for general application is 2 drops each of Lavender, Rosemary, Pine needles, Winter green, Juniper berry and Eucalyptus, prepared in one table spoon of suitable carrier oil.

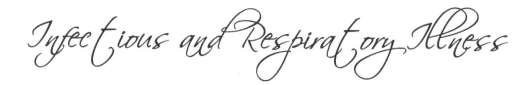
Infectious and Respiratory Illness

ASTHMA AND HAYFEVER

Asthma, characterized by attacks of wheezing and shortness of breath, is very often an allergy-induced disorder, starting in childhood and frequently going hand in hand with bronchitis, hay fever and other allergic reactions such as eczema. An attack can be triggered by an infection like a cold or by allergens such as pollen or dust, but is largely related to over-exertion and stress, especially in those of a nervous disposition.

Hay fever is due to an allergic reaction to pollen or other irritants, and since some essential oils can induce allergic reactions, extreme care must be taken in the choice of a suitable remedy. The following combinations can help to alleviate the problem, but because asthma and hay fever affect people in different ways, the treatment is often a case of trial and error.

*The most useful oil for hay fever and asthma is peppermint, since it is antispasmodic (soothing), expectorant and helps to clear the head. Use regularly in the bath (3 drops only) also use in a vaporizer or on the pillow.

*Oral ingestion of Evening Primrose oil helps boost immune system, regulates body's physiological functions and control allergic reactions.

*Other soothing oils, such as Bergamot, Clary sage, Frankincense, Lavender, Neroli and Mandarin can all help to ease nervous tension or anxiety: add 5-10 drops to the bath water or Vaporize.

*Regular massage, especially on chest and back, using a relaxing, soothing blend can help prevent tension and anxiety building up. A recommended mixture is 2 drops each of Frankincense, Thyme, Rosemary and Lavender in 1 tablespoon carrier oil.

During an attack of asthma and hay fever, those who suffer, can put the following oils on a tissue to inhale: 3 drops in total of Peppermint, Frankincense, Cajeput or Rosemary (or a combination of these).

*For everyday use, add a few drops of Frankincense, Geranium, Lavender and Eucalyptus to a vaporizer to create a relaxing atmosphere in the home.

FLU, COMMON COLDS AND SINUSITIS

The two most useful oils for stimulating the immune system and fighting the cold virus are Eucalyptus and Tea tree. Combine them with Lemon (limonene in Lemon oil boost the antiviral properties of Eucalyptus oil) and Frankincense. At the first sign of a cold appearing, use these oils in a vaporizer or apply a few drops to the pillow or a tissue for inhalation throughout the day and night.

*For shivers, headaches and aching muscles take a warm bath with 3-5 drops each of Lavender, Basil, Ginger and Marjoram. This will also encourage restful sleep.

*Eucalyptus, Rosemary, Lemon, Basil, Peppermint and Bergamot help to reduce temperature and fight infection. A few drops of these oils can be used in a vaporizer or added to a dish of steaming water placed on a radiator in the sick room.

*The best way to combat congestion, sinusitis and catarrh is to use steam inhalations. Add a few drops of Rosemary, Peppermint or Eucalyptus to a bowl of hot water and inhale deeply for 3-10 minutes, keeping eyes closed. In addition, use the above oils in a vaporizer or add a few drops to a tissue for inhalation throughout the day.

*To further clear the head of stuffiness and help fight viral infection add 3 drops each of Rosemary, Peppermint and Lavender, or cajuput with Pine needle to a steaming bath.

*For a sore throat, add 3 drops in total of Clary sage, Sandalwood, Tea tree or Geranium (or a combination of these) to a glass of warm boiled water, with a little fresh lemon juice (an excellent antiseptic). Mix well and gargle. (Not to be used by children under five).

COUGHS AND BRONCHITIS

Coughs can be dry and irritating or they can be accompanied by mucus discharge, especially in association with a cold or with bronchitis.

Bronchitis indicates an inflammation of the bronchial tubes, accompanied by coughing and an over-production of mucus. Acute bronchitis usually starts with a cold or sore throat, which then develops into a fever that lasts a few days. Chronic bronchitis is a long-term condition, without fever, which is aggravated by smoking, a damp climate, air pollution and poor nutrition (especially too many dairy products).

*When there is fever resent, eucalyptus, tea tree, thyme, peppermint and bergamot help to reduce temperature and fight infection. A few drops of these oils can be used in a vaporizer or added to a dish of steaming water placed on a radiator in the sick room.

*The best way to combat excess mucus, congestion and catarrh is to use steam inhalations. Add a few drops of rosemary, peppermint or eucalyptus (or a combination of these) to a bowl of hot water and inhale deeply for 3-10 minutes, keeping the eyes closed. In addition, add a few drops to a tissue for inhalation throughout the day.

*There are many essential oils with balsamic properties which are soothing and help to loosen mucus (for dry or irritating coughs), the most effective being Rosemary, Myrtle, Eucalyptus, Myrrh, Frankincense, Holy Basil, Sandalwood and Pine needle. A few drops of any of these oils can be used in a vaporizer or added to the bath water.

*A local back and chest massage oil, which is effective against bronchitis, coughs and catarrh, can be made by blending 2 drops each of Eucalyptus, Juniper berry, Thyme, Frankincense and Ginger with 1 tablespoon Olive oil. Alternatively, for a dry cough simply add 3 drops each of Pine needle, Holy Basil, Eucalyptus and Atlas Cedarwood to 1 tablespoon of base oil.

*A useful oil for nightly coughs, in children and adults is Myrtle, since it helps to fight infection but it is not too stimulating, which might otherwise prevent sleep. Use a few drops on the pillow or on night clothes or in a vaporizer.

FEVER AND INFECTION

Although essential oils can help provide relief during an infectious illness, as well as reduce its duration and prevent it from spreading in ceases of high fever, severe infection or an acute childhood illness, the following home treatments should not be used as a substitute for professional help.

*The two most useful oils for stimulating the immune system and fighting viruses of all kinds, including flu are eucalyptus and tea tree. Use these oils in a vaporizer in the sick room or put a few drops on the pillow or on a hankie for use throughout the day and night.

*For shivers, headaches and aching muscles take a warm bath with 4 drops each of Lavender, Ginger and Marjoram. This will also encourage restful sleep. Roman chamomile is helpful in overcoming anxiety or insomnia.

*When there is fever present, Eucalyptus, Tea tree, Lemon, Thyme, Ppeppermint and Bergamot help to reduce temperature and fight infection. A few drops of these oils can be used in a vaporizer or added to a dish of steaming water placed on a radiator in the sick room.

*For a sore throat, add 2 drops in total of Clary sage, Spanish sage, Sandalwood, Tea tree or Geranium (and a little fresh lemon juice) to a glass of warm boiled water, mix well and gargle. (Not to be used by children under five).

MOUTH, TOOTH AND GUM INFECTIONS

*A traditional remedy for toothache is to put 1 drop of clove oil on to a cotton-bud and apply to the tooth. (Do not swallow).

*Disease of gums (gingivitis) is a common cause of tooth loss, and care of the gums is vital to health. A good mouth rinse to prevent bleeding or swollen gums is 3 drops in total of Cypress, Clove, Tea Tree, Lemon, Sandalwood, Spanish sage or Thyme (or a combination of any three of these) in a cup of warm boiled water together with a pinch of sea salt. If the infection is severe, a few drops of neat Myrrh should be massaged on to the affected area.

*To treat mouth ulcers, dry the affected area and dab twice daily with Tea Tree or Myrrh. You can use the same oils along with Juniper or Cypress, in warm water for gargles..

*For swelling and pain resulting from infected gums or wisdom teeth, mix 3 drops in total of Clove, Tea Tree and Cypress in 1 teaspoon carrier oil, and massage into the cheeks. A cold compress also helps ease pain.

*A good remedy for bad breath or halitosis is to use the following mixture regularly: 100 ml of cheap brandy or vodka, 10 drops each of Lemon and Peppermint or Spearmint with 5 drops each of Myrrh, Tea tree and Juniper berry. To use, mix 2 or 3 teaspoons in half a cup of warm water, and rinse the mouth out twice daily.

Stress Related Conditions

With the present-day emphasis on materialism and the achievement of external goals, it is important to keep in touch with ourselves on an inner level. Allowing space for ourselves is something that many of us find difficult, whether because of work or through family pressures. Stress is the modern-day disease, and one we all suffer from, at some time or another. When we are stressed we become less resistant to all kinds of illness that affect the body, the emotions and the mind. A lot of modern illnesses are called psychosomatic in origin, in a sense starting at mental level and finally showing in the physical body.

The use of aromatics can help to lift anxiety and bring about a change in our state of mind. This is one of the most traditional uses of essential oils, and the reason they have played an important role in both religious and spiritual rituals for thousands of years. Engaging in the ritual of a candlelit aromatic bath, or burning essences to create a relaxed atmosphere in a room, or using essential oils for massage or to aid mediation, are all ways of slowing down the mind and of becoming more attuned to the moment. It is also important, of course, to try to deal with the causes of stress directly, and if necessary to seek professional help.

Because of the emotional elements which are at play in stress-related conditions, the choice of essential oils depends largely on the causes of the problem, and the temperament of each individual and how they respond under pressure. The following aromatic recipes may provide a few ideas.

DEPRESSION AND ANXIETY

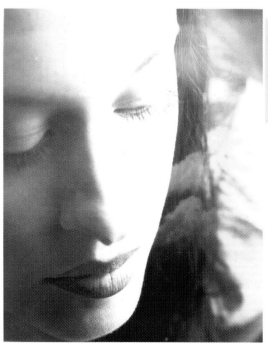

Depression can take many forms, and it is important to try to understand the causes and deal with them directly. Essential oils can help alleviate the symptoms, but since this is primarily an emotional complaint, the method of treatment is very much an individual matter.

*If the depression is associated with lethargy and lack of energy, oils such as sweet/ holy Basil, Bergamot, Geranium, Rosemary, Neroli, Jasmine and Rose can be uplifting and energizing. These can be used in the bath, in a vaporizer, or as perfumes. Practicing massage either on oneself or with a friend can be of great benefit, combining both the comforting effect of touch and the remedial effect of the oils.

*If the depression is associated with restlessness and anxiety, then the more sedating and soothing oils such as

Chamomile, Clary sage, Lavender, Atlas Cedarwood, Marjoram, Vertiver, Ylang ylang and Sandalwood can help encourage a relaxed state of mind. Aromatic bathing massage, scenting the home and using these oils as perfumes, are all ways of bringing enjoyment and pleasure both to the individual and to those around them.

Jasmine and Melissa, along with all citrus oils have been found to be good anti depressants. The oils which have traditionally been used as incenses, such as Benzoin, Atlas Cedarwood, Patchauli, Frankincense, Juniper and Sandalwood, can help bring about a calm state of mind, used either as perfumes or in a vaporizer. Since there are so many oils to choose from when it comes to helping depression, one of the best ways of deciding is simply to select the scent which appeals and gives a lift to the emotions in that moment.

DIGESTIVE UPSETS

Digestive upsets are often the result of stored anxieties. They respond well to the external application of essential oils, but this is often enhanced by the use of herbal remedies, such as peppermint, chamomile or fennel tea.

*Stomach ache of nervous origin can be helped by gentle massage to the abdomen, especially in the area of solar plexus, in a clockwise direction using 9 drops in total of Marjoram, Rosemary, Lavender, Fennel or Thyme (or a combination of these) in 1 tablespoon carrier oil. Neroli is also soothing in cases of nerves or emotional upsets, used in the bath, as vaporized oil or in a massage combination.

*For indigestion with wind, use 9 drops in total of Fennel or spearmint (or a combination of both) in 1 tablespoon carrier oil for abdominal massage (clockwise) as indicated above.

*To help ease constipation, use 9 drops in total of Rosemary, Thyme, Fennel seed (or a combination of these) in 1 tablespoon carrier oil for abdominal massage (Clockwise).

*If there is diarrhea or a viral infection is suspected, use 9 drops in total of Tea tree, Juniper, Oregano and Thyme (or a combination of these) in 1 tablespoon carrier oil for massage as indicated above. A warm bath with 4 drops each of Juniper, Thyme and 2 drops of ginger is also recommended.

The other spice oils are also very beneficial to help relieve pain and promote digestion, used in minute amounts in massage oils or baths. They include Black pepper, Carrot seed, Clove, Cardamom, Cinnamon, Coriander and Ginger.

FATIGUE, POOR CIRCULATION AND LOW BLOOD PRESSURE (HYPOTENSION)

Fatigue can be caused by exhaustion and stress, or can be related to feelings of lethargy due to a slow metabolic rate. Poor circulation and low blood pressure, often occur together, and in both cases stimulating essences are advised. Attention to diet and exercise is also very beneficial, especially for those with a sedentary lifestyle.

*Rosemary is the most useful oil for this condition, being stimulating and tonic. Use 5-10 drops of Black Pepper and Rosemary, or 3-5 drops of Peppermint with sweet/holy Basil or Petitgrain and Sage in the bath.

*A vigorous massage using 5 drops of Rosemary, 2 drops Lemongrass or Melissa along with 2 drops of Black pepper in 1 tablespoon carrier oil also helps to stimulate the system.

*Exhaustion and fatigue of a more emotional nature can be helped by mentally reviving and uplifting oils such as Jasmine, Basil, Bergamot, Neroli, Melissa or Geranium, used in vaporizers or as perfumes.

*Excessive fatigue can be counteracted with refreshing and uplifting bath oils which may be used in the morning or before going out in the evening after a heavy day. Recommended bath blends are 3-5 drops each of Rosemary, Geranium, Mandarin and Basil, or Rosemary, Melissa with Petitgrain, or a combination of Geranium, Neroli, and sweet basil

HEADACHES AND MIGRAINE

For tension headaches apply neat Lavender to the temples or to the back of the neck; to ease strain and tension, massage the shoulders and neck using 1 teaspoon carrier oil with 3 drops in total of Lavender, Basil or Marjoram (or a combination of both).

*For congested headaches due to blocked sinuses, use a few drops of Peppermint with Eucalyptus, on a tissue to inhale throughout the day, you can also use these oils in a vaporizer or added to a bowl of steaming water as an inhalation.

Migraine is most commonly a food-related complaint, but an attack can also be triggered by an increase in stress or anxiety. A cold compress placed on the temples using 1 drop of Lavender and Peppermint, can help to case discomfort during an attack. As a preventive measure, soothing and relaxing oils such as Lavender, Roman chamomile, Basil, Marjoram, Neroli and Sandalwood should be used on a daily basis in baths, massages, vaporizers or as perfumes.

HIGH BLOOD PRESSURE (HYPERTENSION)

Although aromatherapy treatments have been found to reduce blood pressure significantly, it is vital also to review issues such as diet, exercise and general lifestyle. In addition, garlic, either eaten raw or taken as pearls or tablets, has been found to help reduce cholesterol and control high blood pressure. Stimulants, such as tea, coffee and alcohol, should be reduced or eliminated. Evening primrose oil taken orally 1 teaspoon daily with Lacithin also helps to regularize blood pressure.

*Regular massage is particularly helpful for this condition and can dramatically reduce high blood pressure - an excellent blend for massage at home is 3 drops each of Ylang Ylang, Lavender, Clary sage and Marjoram in 2 tablespoons carrier oil.

*The use of other relaxing and sedative oils such as bergamot, Roman Chamomile, Patchouli, Vertiver or Sandalwood is also effective. Use 5-10 drops of any of these oils (or a combination of them) in the bath, in a vaporizer or as a perfume.

*5-10 drops of any of the cleansing and detoxifying oils, which include Fennel, Grapefruit and Juniper with Lavender and Ylang Ylang, are also beneficial when used in the bath (or for massage).

NERVOUS TENSION AND INSOMNIA

For the workaholics, some good soothing bath combinations to use before retiring are 2-3 drops each of Lavender, Vertiver or Sandal with Roman Chamomile and Patchouli. Other oils which are also very beneficial for relaxation are Geranium, Clary sage, Ylang ylang and Atlas Cedarwood.

*Emotional stress and nervous tension expresses itself in different ways, some people cope by becoming over-active, some people become depressed, while others collapse. Some good basic bath combinations which are supportive and comforting are 3-5 drops each of Bergamot, Geranium and Neroli (anti-depressant), or Sandalwood, Lavender and Geranium (soothing, Relaxing), or Jasmine, Ylang Ylang and Geranium (uplifting and stimulating).

*A full body massage at the hands of a qualified aromatherapist, can do much to alleviate stress, but massage can also be carried out in the home. A recommended blend for general tension/ irritability is 3 drops each of Lavender, Geranium, Ylang ylang and Clary sage in 2 tablespoon (30 ml) carrier oil.

*Tension is often held in the body, especially in the neck and shoulder areas. A good massage blend, for easing muscular tension and general aches and pains in 3 drops of Rosemary, Marjoram, Lavender or a combination of these in 1 tablespoon (15ml) of suitable base oil.

*The best oils for the insomnia that often accompanies stress are Lavender, Clary Sage, Marjoram, Roman Chamomile and Patchauli. Use in the bath, or put a few drops on the pillow or in a vaporizer in the bedroom before retiring.

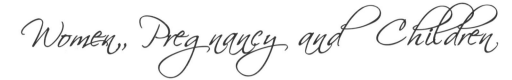
Women, Pregnancy and Children

CELLULITE

Although aromatherapy is very successful in helping to combat cellulite, this obviously needs to be supported by exercise, dietary measures and, if possible, professional lymphatic massage (which encourages elimination of toxins via the lymphatic system). Hormonal imbalance, as well as stress and too much tea, coffee and alcohol, which all increase toxicity levels, also contribute to this condition.

These stimulating, toxin-eliminating bath oil blends should be used on successive days: 3-4 drops each of Rosemary, Juniper, Lemon grass and Grapefruit. They can also be applied to a loofah or massage glove and rubbed into the affected areas while bathing.

*A good detoxifying massage oil can be made by blending 2 drops each of Rosemary, Geranium and Juniper along with 1 drop of Lemongrass & Orange with 1 tablespoon of chosen carrier oil.

*General massage also helps to improve the circulation as well as reduce cellulite. Oils such as Cypress, Thyme, Spanish sage, Rosemary and Mandarin are also of beneficial in this case.

CYSTITIS AND PRURITIS (ITCHING)

Cystitis, which is an infection of the bladder, is characterized by a painful burning sensation while passing urine. Pruritis, or itching, is an irritating condition which often accompanies a mild vaginal infection. Take garlic pearls, drink plenty of water and keep tea, coffee, alcohol and spices to a minimum. Avoid tight-fitting clothes and nylon underwear.

*For Cystitis, make up a solution (well shaken) using 5 drops each of Tea Tree, German chamomile. Sandalwood and Bergamot in 1 pint of cooled boiled water. Using a piece of soaked cotton wool, swab the opening of the urethra frequently (if possible, each time after passing urine).

*In addition make up a massage oil, using 3 drops each of German chamomile, Bergamot, Tea tree, Sandalwood and Lavender with I tablespoon carrier oil. This blend should be massaged into the lower back and abdomen twice daily.

*To help combat cystitis and pruritis, it is beneficial to bathe frequently using bactericidal essential oils. Add 5-10 drops of a combination containing Lavender, German chamomile, Juniper, Sandalwood, Tea tree to a warm bath, or add 2-3 drops to a bidet for local washing.

MENSTRUAL PROBLEMS

Essential oils can help to combat menstrual disorders on a variety of levels, because they are able to operate on the emotional and the physical sides simultaneously. One of the most useful oil for all kinds of menstrual problems is Clary sage.

*For period pains, gently massage the lower abdomen and lower back with the following blend containing 9 drops of Lavender, Clary sage and Marjoram in 1 tablespoon base oil.
Alternatively, add a few drops of Clary sage and Marjoram to a hot compress, and apply to the abdomen.

*The effects of pre-menstrual tension can be eased by taking regular aroma baths, with oils which help to relieve tension. Add 5-10 drops of either Lavender, Clary sage, Neroli or Rose to the bath water. In chronic cases 1 teaspoonful Evening Primrose oil, taken orally, for a period of three months helps a lot.

*To help regulate heavy flow, make a massage oil blend using 9 drops of Cypress, Geranium and Clary sage, in 1 tablespoon carrier oil and rub anticlockwise, on lower abdomen. In addition you can use 5-10 drops of these oils in the bath. Diet, exercise and emotional factors should also be assessed.

*To help promote or normalize scanty menstruation, make a massage oil blend, using 9 drops total, of Clary sage, Juniper berry and Roman chamomile in 1 tablespoon carrier oil to rub clockwise on lower abdomen. In addition you can use 5-10 drops of these oils in the bath. Diet (poor diet, anemia and being run down often accompany this problem) other lifestyle factors should also be assessed.

EDEMA (WATER RETENTION)

Although this is not an exclusively female complaint, edema often occurs during the later stages of pregnancy. It may also be caused by being overweight or other factors such as food allergies, standing for long periods or hormonal imbalance. It most commonly occurs in legs around ankles and knees; but can also be found in the hands, stomach, or around the eyes.

*The most useful oils are Juniper Berry, Fennel, Geranium and Rosemary. Add 9 drops of a combination of these to 1 tablespoon carrier oil or cream and massage gently at the site of the swelling. Legs should be massaged with upward strokes.

*Alternatively, massage the soles of the feet with 2-3 drops each of Juniper berry, Cypress and Lavender, in 1 tablespoon carrier oil.

*For swollen ankles, submerge in a lukewarm footbath containing a few drops of Juniper Berry, Cypress, Fennel, Geranium or Rosemary.

*Take warm baths containing 5-10 drops of the aforesaid oils combination.

*Swelling and puffiness can also be relieved by applying a cold compress using 1 teaspoon Witch hazel lotion with 2 drops each of Juniper and German chamomile to the affected area.

THRUSH (CANDIDA) AND LEUCORRHOEA

Thrush is a form of fungal infection, which affects warm, moist parts of the body, but most commonly occurs in the vagina, where symptoms include itching and a thick milky discharge.

Leucorrhoea is an inflammation of the vagina caused by the proliferation of unwanted fungi, resulting in a thick white or yellow discharge.

Both conditions are aggravated by tight clothing, nylon underwear, harsh bubble baths, and the use of antibiotics. Most cases of thrush and leucorrhoea respond well to the use of Tea tree oil.

*Add 5-10 drops of Tea tree to the bath water daily (check sensitivity first) or a few drops to a sitz bath for a local wash.

*Make a douche by mixing 10 drops of Tea tree with 1 pint of cooled boiled water and bathe the area using an enema pot, or soak a tampon in the above solution and insert into the vagina.

*Other oils of benefit which may be used in the bath include Geranium, Juniper, Lavender, Oregano and Bergamot: add 5-10 drops to the bath water.

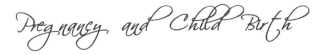

Pregnancy and Child Birth

PREPARING FOR MOTHERHOOD

More and more women wish to deliver their baby in as natural and as active a way possible, without the use of drugs. There are now many books available on the subject, which cover issues such as nutrition, exercise or herbal remedies (for example, raspberry tea), all of which can help to make pregnancy and the birth easier and more enjoyable. Essential oils are being used increasingly by nurses and midwives in this context.

Using essential oils during pregnancy to help with childbirth can be very beneficial in a variety of ways, but there are some precautions to be taken, due to the sensitivity of the womb and the unborn foetus.

1. Use all essential oils at half the usual stated amount during pregnancy.

2. The oils which should be avoided altogether are Basil, Cinnamon, Citronella, Clary sage, Clove, Hyssop, Juniper, Marjoram, Myrrh, Spanish sage, Tarragon and Thyme.

3. The oils which are best avoided during the first four months of pregnancy are Cedar wood, Fennel, Peppermint and Rosemary.

PREGNANCY

*An excellent oil to help prevent stretch marks can be made by blending 2 drops each of Lavender and Palmarosa with 1 drop each of Neroli and Frankincense added to 1 teaspoon wheat germ plus 1 tablespoon Olive oil - for light massage daily to the belly and breasts. This oil can also help to lighten existing stretch marks.

*In addition, Wheatgerm oil can also be rubbed into the perineum to help prepare for the birth. Research has shown that massaging the perineum for 5-10 minutes daily in the last six weeks of pregnancy can help prevent tearing.

*Aromatic bathing offers great pleasure and relief, especially towards the end of pregnancy. Add 3-5 drops of any of the following oils to the bath: uplifting oils like Bergamot, Neroli, Mandarin, Geranium and Jasmine or relaxing oils like Sandalwood, Rose, Lavender, Patchouli, Ylang ylang, Frankincense etc.
*Pamper yourself during pregnancy, using the following essential oils as perfumes or as soothing air fresheners to overcome anxiety and encourage a relaxed attitude to the forthcoming birth - Lavender to

relax, Roman chamomile, Vertiver or Sandal to calm the mind, Bergamot, Neroli and Mandarin to uplift, rose or jasmine to comfort.

*Gentle massage can be very enjoyable during pregnancy, and can help with a wide variety of problems, such a back pain. To soothe back pain and relax the body, lie on one side and ask a friend or partner to use the following blend, applied to the lower back: 3 drops each of Lavender and Roman chamomile in I tablespoon of nourishing base oil.

*Edema, fatigue, varicose veins, constipation and other digestive problems are also common during pregnancy (refer to respective ailment). Always take care to avoid contra-indicated oils, and use in low dilutions only.

LABOUR

A traditional and useful massage oil to help prepare for the birth and strengthen the uterus muscles is to blend 2 drops of Jasmine with 1 drop of Nutmeg in 1 teaspoon of nourishing base carrier oil. Rub the oil on to the lower abdomen each day, for two weeks prior to the expected delivery.

During the birth and in preparing to bring the baby into the home the use of vaporized oils to scent the environment can create an uplifting, relaxed mood. They also prevent the spread of airborne bacteria. Use a few drops of Lavender, Frankincense, Mandarin or Bergamot in a vaporizer, or in a bowl of hot water on a radiator.

Pain relief during labor can be aided by firm massage to the lower back using the following blend: 3 drops of Lavender, 2 drops each of Geranium and Rosemary in 1 tablespoon carrier oil.

AFTER THE DELIVERY

*To help heal the perineum after the birth, add 2 drops of Cypress and 3 drops of Lavender to a shallow bath, and soak. Repeat each day. This also helps to prevent infection.

*It is common to feel many mixed emotions after the birth. Post-natal depression can be helped by the use of uplifting and comforting oils, such as Lavender, Bergamot, Jasmine, Rose and Neroli. Geranium and Clary sage can help to normalize; hormonal imbalance and regulate mood swings. Use in the bath, for massage or in vaporizers.

*Engorged breasts can be soothed using a cold compress, or through gentle massage using 2-3 drops of Juniper and Fennelseed oil to 1 tablespoon base oil or cream.

*For sore nipples, blend 1 drop of Rose, Sandalwood, Lavender in 1 teaspoon of non-oily cream or gel between feeds. Wipe off using a bland cream before each feed or use squeezed Lemon peel for wiping nipples.

NOTE: Calendula or chamomile ointments are also useful soothing remedies for cracked nipples.

Babies, Infants and Children

BABIES AND INFANTS

Babies and infants respond especially well to natural healing methods, but their extra sensitivity must be taken into account. Do not attempt to substitute a home remedy for professional treatment if it is needed.

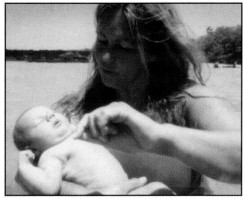

*Babies 0-12 months: Use only 1 drop of, either Lavender, Rose, Roman Chamomile, Neroli or Geranium essential oil, diluted in 1 teaspoon carrier oil for massage or bathing.

*Infants 1-5 years: Use only 2-3 drops of the 'safe' essential oils as above, diluted in 1 teaspoon carrier oil for massage or bathing, avoid all those oils which are potentially toxic or which may cause skin irritation. See 'Safety Guidelines' to know for which oils to avoid.

OLDER CHILDREN

Older children enjoy the stimulation of different scents. By the age of six they can recognize a wide range of smells, and enjoy being introduced to new experiences. It is fun to choose an oil to put in the bath or use as a scent. Geranium and Lavender are popular with children because they are familiar and sweet. Add about 5 drops to the bath at bedtime.

*Children 6-12 years: Use as for adults but in half the stated concentration.

*Teenagers: Use as directed for adults.

COMMON CHILDHOOD COMPLAINTS

Many common childhood complaints can be treated with essential oils. Always check the dilution with the guidelines above.

*Nappy rash in babies and infants can be prevented by regular bathing using 1 drop of either Lavender or Roman/ German chamomile diluted in 1 teaspoon carrier oil. If nappy rash does occur add 1 drop each of Tea tree with Lavender or Roman/ German chamomile to 1 teaspoon of a non/greasy baby cream and apply gently at each nappy change: Nappy rash is often caused by thrush.

*Restlessness and insomnia in babies, infants and older children can be helped by the use of Lavender, Rose, Roman/ German chamomile or Neroli, in the bath or for massage. Alternatively, use a vaporizer in the bedroom (ensure it is out of children's reach), or put a drop or two of oil on the pillow or on the pajamas suit.

*Tummy ache and colic in babies, infants and older children can be eased by 1-3 drops of Lavender, Marjoram and Roman chamomile in 1 teaspoon carrier oil gently massaged to the lower back or stomach in a clockwise direction.

*Teething pain in babies and infants can be relieved by mixing 1 drop of Roman chamomile and Lavender in 1 teaspoon of carrier oil and massaging into the check.

*For cuts, spots, insect bites and other skin blemishes for infants over one year old, apply 1 drop of neat lavender.

INFECTIOUS ILLNESSES

The most useful oil for stimulating the immune system and fighting viruses of all kinds in children, including flu, chickenpox and measles, is Tea tree. A few drops of Tea tree, Lavender and Frankincense should be used in a vaporizer or put on the pillow or on a hankie for use throughout the day and night.

For fever and whooping cough add a few drops of Basil and Bergamot to a vaporizer or in a dish of steaming water placed on a radiator in the sick room. Steam vaporizations are especially useful during whooping cough to help relieve the coughing.

*Colds and coughs in infants and older children respond well to the use of essential oils. Put a drop or two of a combination of Myrtle, Marjoram, Cedar wood and Tea tree on the pillow or on the pajamas suit. You can also mix 3 drops of this combination to 1 teaspoon olive oil. Alternatively, use a few drops of any of the above oils in a vaporizer in the bedroom (ensure it is well out of reach).

*For infants and children add 2-4 drops of Lavender and Geranium or Mandarin to the bath at the first signs of a cold developing.

*To help reduce itching and prevent scarring from chickenpox, make a lotion using 50ml Witch hazel, 50ml Rosewater, with 2 drops each of German chamomile, Tea tree and Lavender and dab on to the blisters. If the child is under five, add up to 3 drops of Lavender or German chamomile to a warm bath with a handful of colloidal oatmeal (available from some chemists) and soak for 10 minutes at least twice a day.

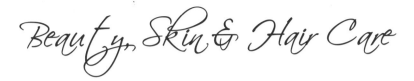

SKIN AND HAIR CARE

Essential oils are ideally suited to skin care, for they are readily absorbed and have the ability to penetrate through to the underlying layers of the skin, which are alive and active, unlike the outer dead layer of cells that are constantly being shed. Essential oils stimulate cellular regeneration, improve the circulation and help to eliminate toxins at a fundamental level. Skin that has been treated with aromatic oils thus becomes more dynamic and healthy. In addition, because the oils are able to travel in the bloodstream and lymphatic system, skin treatments using essential oils are vitalizing to the body as a whole.

ACNE AND SPOTS

This common skin complaint is caused by over-activity of the sebaceous glands, and is most common during adolescence, the menopause and at times of hormonal imbalance or change, such as before menstruation. Poor diet, lack of exercise, stress and anxiety can further aggravate the condition. It has already been discussed in detail earlier in chapter covering body parts "FACE".

*Apply an aromatic flower water, as a toner/cleanser to the skin morning and evening. To prepare, mix 25ml witch hazel, 75ml rosewater with 5 drops each of Lemon, Tea tree, Geranium and Lavender. Let it mature for up to a month, and then filter before use with coffee filter paper. (It is a good idea to prepare a whole batch in one go).

*Use a light facial oil, containing 2 teaspoons sweet almond oil, 1 teaspoon wheat germ oil 1 tea spoon Borage or Evening primrose as base to which you add 3 drops each of Palmarosa, Juniper, Tea tree and Lavender (remove excess with cotton wool). Individual spots can be dabbed with neat lavender or tea tree (check sensitization first).

*A good facial mask can be made by mixing 2 tablespoons of green clay, 1 teaspoon of jojoba oil, 1 teaspoon of yoghurt, with 3 drops each of Juniper and Palmarosa oil.

*To help unclog the pores of the skin, put 3 drops each of Juniper and Geranium in a bowl of steaming water as a facial steam. Putting pine needle oil or Lavender mixed with water on the stove when having a sauna has a similar effect on the whole body.

*3-5 drops each of Lavender and Palmarosa, or Juniper and Rosemary, or Petitgrain and Geranium may be added to the bath water to help detoxify the body. This also acts as a kind of facial steam.

*Shaving spots or barber's rash can be helped by the following lotion: 100ml orange flower water and 1 teaspoon vodka to which has been added 5 drops each of Tea tree and sandalwood oil. Shake the mixture well before use.

*Regular body massage (by a friend, partner or by a professional), using 3 drops each of Geranium, Juniper and Rosemary in 1 tablespoon basic carrier oil, will also help to stimulate the lymphatic system and rid the body of toxins.

AGEING SKIN, THREAD VEINS AND WRINKLES

Ageing is inevitable, but essential oils can do much to slow down the effects. They encourage regeneration of healthy cells and help to keep the skin supple and elastic. General lifestyle is also, of course, very important, since smoking, drugs, poor diet, too much sun, and heat and stress can all speed up the ageing process. (For details please check the chapter on body parts- Face.)

*The regular use of facial oil containing cytophylactic oils (those that stimulate new cell growth and prevent wrinkles) is vital. They are Lavender, Neroli, Frankincense, Geranium, Rose and Sandalwood. Add 3 drops of any of these oils to 1 teaspoon wheat germ oil, for gentle application, especially to the area around the eyes, before retiring.

*A good basic blend for the face and neck is as follows: 1 tablespoon Jojoba oil, 1 teaspoon Wheat germ oil, 6 drops of lavender, 3 drops of Geranium and 2 drops of Frankincense. An extra teaspoon of a rich carrier oil such apricot kernel, avocado, hazelnut, evening primrose or peach kernel may also be added.

*Gentle facial massage, avoiding the delicate area around the eyes, helps to improve circulation and muscle tone. Use the following blend: 1 tablespoon jojoba and 1 teaspoon Evening primrose oil with 9 drops in total of Rose, Sandalwood, Rosewood or Palmarosa (or a combination of these).

*A face mask made by mixing 2 tablespoons clay, 2 teaspoons runny honey, 1 teaspoon water and 4 drops of Rose or Geranium oil, used once a week, helps rejuvenation.

*Thread veins and broken capillaries are best treated, using a facial oil employing 3 drops of Roman chamomile or Rose in 1 teaspoon jojoba oil.

DRY AND SENSITIVE SKIN

Dry skin becomes wrinkled more easily than greasy skin and needs to be moisturized and nourished regularly, especially when exposed to the effects of sun and wind.

For a moisturizing treatment on dry skin, add 9 drops in total of Sandalwood, Geranium and Vertiver to 1 tablespoon of Jojoba with 1 teaspoon of a rich oil, such as Avocado, Borage, Evening Primrose or Wheat germ, and apply daily. Remove excess with a cotton wool pad.

*A good toner/cleanser for dry skin can be made by adding 5 drops each of Lavender, Geranium and Vertiver to 75ml Rosewater, letting it stand for up to a month before filtering. Then add 25 ml glycerine and shake well. Use twice daily.

*For moisturizing sensitive skin, it is important to avoid all possible irritants and to use only the gentlest essences- Roman chamomile, Lavender, Neroli, Sandalwood and Rose are the best choice. Add 5 drops of any of the above oils to 1 tablespoon of jojoba, apricot or peach kernel oil or an anti-allergenic cream or lotion for daily use.

*An excellent basic purifying and rejuvenating face mask for dry and sensitive skin can be made by mixing 2 tablespoons of fuller's earth, 2 teaspoons cornflower, 1 egg yolk, 1 teaspoon evening primrose oil (or other rich vegetable oil) with 1 drop each of Geranium, Sandalwood and Rose. Leave on the skin, for 15 minutes, then rinse off, with cool water. (Also see the chapter on Face care)

GREASY AND COMBINATION SKIN

Oily skin is prone to spots and blackheads. It requires careful attention with regard to hygiene and it is also important not to strip the skin of its protective mantle which maintains the natural pH balance.

*Add 3 drops each of Lavender, Geranium and Sandalwood, to 1 tablespoon of any light carrier oil, such as Grape seed with Jojoba, and massage into the skin before retiring for the night. Take care to remove all traces of the oil from the face with a tissue or with cotton wool.

*A good toner/cleanser for greasy or combination skin is to mix 5 drops each of Petitgrain, Lavender and Geranium with 25ml witch hazel and 75ml orange flower water. Let it stand for up to a month then filter. Apply twice daily.

*An excellent basic purifying and rejuvenating face mask for greasy and combination skin can be made by mixing 2 tablespoons green clay, 2 teaspoons cornflower, 1 egg yolk, 1 teaspoon Evening Primrose oil with 1 drop each of Geranium and Lavender. Leave on the skin for 15 minutes, and then rinse off with cool water.

*Add 5-10 drops of Lemon, Palmarosa, Rosewood, Grapefruit, Petitgrain and Geranium to the bath. This also acts as a facial steam.

HAIR CARE

Since our hair is such a vital feature of our appearance it is important to keep it as healthy as possible. Essential oils can be used in several ways to enhance different hair types.

A few drops (approximately 1 per cent) of an essential oil suited to your hair type can be added to your shampoo- it is always better to use a mild or pH neutral shampoo which does not strip the hair of its protective acid mantle. For greasy hair, use Rosemary or Juniper; for dry hair Cedarwood and Patchouli; for fair hair Ylang ylang and Palmarosa; and for dark hair atlas cedarwood and Ylang ylang.

For a good rinse for all hair types, add 5 drops of Rosemary or Lemon essential oil, together with 1 tablespoon cider vinegar to the final rinse. This will also help to remove detergent residue and restore the acid equilibrium of the scalp.

*The following conditioning treatment is excellent for all hair types, but especially if the hair is dry or damaged. Mix 2 tablespoons jojoba oil with 30 drops of an essential oil suited to your hair type as mentioned above. Warm the oil slightly and massage into damp hair, then cover with a shower cap and leave on for 2 hours (if possible). Shampoo out, later on.

*Dandruff responds well to Tea tree, Rosemary and Eucalyptus, used in the shampoo and final rinse. Juniper is also very helpful in the conditioning treatment described above.

*An effective tonic, which also promotes hair growth, can be made by mixing 2 tablespoon vodka with 5 drops each of Rosemary, Cedarwood and Ylang Ylang, massage well into the scalp. Other oils which promote hair growth are Spanish sage and Clary sage.

*Lice are a common problem, especially among school children, Lavender, Juniper, Eucalyptus and Tea tree are very effective in ridding the hair of lice and preventing their return. A few drops (1 per cent) should be added to a mild shampoo for regular use, and about 5 drops included in the final rinse. In addition, an alcohol-based treatment can be made by mixing 10 drops of Eucalyptus and 5 drops of tea tree with 1 tablespoon of vodka and massaging into the scalp. (If the skin is irritated, use vegetable oil in place of the vodka).

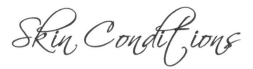

ECZEMA (DERMATITIS) & PSORIASIS

This type of skin condition is characterized by flaky skin, itchy rashes, inflammation and sometimes weeping blisters or scabs. It is frequently associated with hereditary allergic tendencies, but often flares up during times of emotional difficulties or stress. It is important to try to locate the cause of the problem and deal with it directly. This means identifying the type of allergens which aggravate the condition and avoiding them (these may be particular household chemicals, dust, or certain foods); it may also mean looking at the emotional environment and making changes if necessary.

*In general, the most useful oils, for eczema is German chamomile, Juniper and Tea tree, and the best medium is usually a non-allergenic light aqueous cream or gel. You can also add about 6 drops of Tea tree and German Chamomile to 1 tablespoon of cream or gel to make a very dilute ointment, and apply at least 3 times daily.

*If the condition is weepy or inflamed, 2 drops of Myrrh or Patchouli should be included in the above cream or gel.

*If the condition is very itchy, add a few drops of German chamomile, Tea tree and Juniper to a cold compress and apply to the skin. Using a few drops of chamomile or lavender in the bath can also help to alleviate itching. (A handful of powdered or colloidal oatmeal, available from some chemists, is also very soothing when added to the bath water).

Since eczema takes many forms, and is often stress-related, it is helpful to try, to ease emotional tension by using relaxing and uplifting oils such as Lavender, Geranium, Bergamot, Neroli or Rose, for general use in the bath or as room fragrances. Some of my friends, having naturopathy centers, recommend application (twice daily) of self urine on affected area, for at least 15 minutes before you wash it off, according to them it is quite effective for treating chronic skin conditions like, eczema and Psoriasis.

Psoriasis is a common, genetically determined, inflammatory skin disorder of unknown cause, which in its most usual form is characterized by well demarcated raised red scaling patches that preferentially localize to the extensor surfaces. In case of Psoriasis, which sometimes confused with eczema, useful oils are Cade, Juniper, Benzoin, Frankincense, Tea tree and Patchouli. Add 10 drops of any three of these oils in 1 teaspoonful of Jojoba oil for skin application.

Both eczema and psoriasis can be helped greatly with Evening Primrose oil Oral. (Refer to the chapter on Evening Primrose Oil).

ABSCESSES AND BOILS

These often occur when the body is exhausted or run down, at times of hormonal upheaval, and especially if the person is on a poor diet. Always keep the area clean, and treat a boil or abscess before it bursts to avoid the spread of infection.

*Make up a hot compress using clean lint with 2 drops each of Tea tree and Lavender, apply to the affected area; then treat it with one drop of neat Lavender and Tea tree combination, at least 3 times daily, if possible. Cover with a plaster only if necessary.

*A green clay dressing with 1 drop of Tea tree may also be used to help draw out the pus.

*5-10 drops of an antiseptic essential oil can also be added to the bath, such as Bergamot, German chamomile, Geranium, Juniper, Lavender and Tea tree.

ATHLETE'S FOOT AND RINGWORM

These are both contagious fungal infections characterized by red, flaky skin and itching. Athlete's foot occurs between the toes, sometimes affecting the toe nails. Ringworm or Tinea incognito, show on the skin as round, red scaling, well demarcated patches; generally affect the scalp, knees, elbows or between the fingers. Let the skin breathe by avoiding tight clothes and nylon socks.

*Make a blend using 1 teaspoon almond oil, 1drop each of lavender, myrrh and tea tree and apply at least 3 times a day. Tea tree may also be applied neat (or diluted in a gel) - check sensitization first by patch test.

*A few drops of the above oils may also be added to the bath, or to a footbath in the case of athlete's foot.

CHILBLAINS

Injury from cold is well known as frost bite and Chilblains. While frost bite causes acute tissue necrosis of fingers, toes, nose ears, rarely elsewhere; chilblains mostly affect older women, occur at the extremities of the body - fingers and toes mainly due to cold and lack of circulation. Exercise and warm clothing are important preventative factors.

*Apply lemon or tea tree essential oils neat (or diluted in a gel) to the affected area.

*Local blood circulation can be improved by massaging the feet or hands with 2 drops of marjoram and 1 drop of black pepper in 1 teaspoon carrier oil.

COLD SORES AND HERPES

*Mix 3 drops of Tea tree or Chamomile with 1 teaspoon of gel and apply several times daily as soon as the first signs occur. If the skin keeps cracking, alternate the above treatment with German chamomile oil and Lavender 3 drops each in 1 teaspoon Calendula & 1 teaspoon wheat germ oil to keep the area soft.

VARICOSE VEINS AND PILES (HAEMORRHOIDS)

These conditions are both caused by dilated veins brought on by poor circulation and are especially common during pregnancy. Varicose veins occur mainly in the legs; piles or hemorrhoids around the anal area. They both require similar treatments, although sufferers from varicose veins need more patience to see any improvement. The following treatments should be carried out in addition to gentle exercise (inverted yoga postures are especially helpful), keeping weight off the feet as much as possible, improving your diet and losing weight.

*The most useful oils are cypress and geranium: use 5-10 drops in the bath. Other oils of benefit to use in the bath include lavender, juniper and rosemary.

* To make an oil, that will both prevent and alleviate varicose veins, mix 6 drops of geranium and 2 drops of cypress with 1 tablespoon carrier oil (or add to a non-greasy cream). Then use the oil blend to stroke the legs very gently, working upwards from ankle to thigh (do not massage directly on the veins themselves).

*To treat piles, make an ointment by adding 2 drops of myrtle, geranium or cypress to I teaspoon of jelly, and rub around the anal area as required.

VERUCCAE, WARTS AND CORNS

*For these conditions, put a single drop of neat Tea tree on the centre of the verucca, wart or corn every morning and cover with a plaster. It may take several weeks to see any result- but it is effective in the long run. You can also use a combination of Tea Tree with Oregano 15 drops each in one teaspoon of Calendula oil, apply three times daily on the affected area.

PURELY FOR PLEASURE

Experimenting with the aromatic potential of essential oils can be fun. The oils can be blended in infinite combinations to produce individual perfumes, room fragrances, bath essences, etc. To produce a personal fragrance is also a creative and educational experience.

Indian attars were initially designed as therapeutic perfumes, using essential oils as per the season. Certain essential oils like Jasmine, Sandalwood, Rose etc. can be worn straight or diluted in Jojoba as personal perfume or you can blend few oils together to create your signature perfume. The different depths of fragrance in a blend are called 'notes' and each scent takes on a particular character according to the balance of base, middle and top notes from which it has been made. Top notes are those light oils which evaporate quickly, like Lemon, Melissa, Neroli, Bergamot or Grapefruit. The middle notes provide the heart of a blend and include oils like Lavender, Geranium or Rosewood. The heavier base notes linger for hours, and act as the fixative for the other lighter oils. Traditional base notes are viscous oils like Sandalwood, Patchouli, Vertiver, Myrrh and Benzoin. A well-balanced fragrance should contain elements from each group-top, middle and base notes.

APHRODISIACS

Certain oils have the reputation for increasing sexual desire, including Cedarwood, Ylang ylang, Jasmine, Neroli, Patchouli, Rose, Sandalwood Clove and Frankincense. Use 5-10 drops of a combination of three oils in the bath, to create a romantic atmosphere.

*You can also create a combination of aforesaid oils to vaporize in the bedroom to create a sensual mood, or use in your wardrobe to scent linen or clothes, besides protecting them.

*The spice oils, which include Black pepper, Cardamom, Clove, Nutmeg and Ginger, are also reputed to have aphrodisiac properties. However, because they have strong natural chemicals which may cause skin sensitization hence they should be used only in moderation- 3 drops in the bath or 1-2 drops added to other blends.

Evening Primrose Oil

Natures Gift
PANACEA FOR MODERN AILMENTS

Since the time I came to know of evening primrose oil and its multiple benefits, I was wondering, how a single plant oil can be so versatile in its effect. Once I understood the way it works on our body system, my doubts were cleared to quite an extent and I was willing to try the product and was amazed at the results reported to me by my clients. Out of my experience with the oil now I can safely recommend intake of this oil (1 tsp./ 5 ml. daily) to everybody specially women in their thirties or above. Best to ingest this oil for a period of three months after every six months and experience the difference in your health and body energy level.

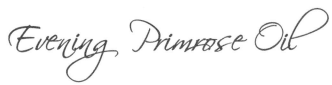

Evening Primrose is an is not a primrose at all, it is related to the rose bay willow herb family, it acquired its name because of its bright yellow primrose look alike flowers and because its flowers open between 6 and 7 o'clock in the evening, when eight or ten of the largest fragrant flower burst open every minute. The flower usually last for whole of next day in dull weather but fade quickly in bright sun light.

Unlike many other natural products known mainly for its therapeutic effect on one condition, the oil of evening primrose has properties, which make it useful for a very wide range of illnesses, from gout, hiccups, breast problems, PMS, blood pressure, faulty blood vessels, brittle nails and score of other ailments just with one gulp.

All these problems seem very different, but evening primrose has something in it which is needed in each one of them. Evening primrose oil is a rich source of essential fatty acids also called vitamin F, because body must have them but can't make them. They are an essential part of nutrition, besides it contains one of the rarest ingredient called GLA (gamma Linolenic Acid) which sets it apart from most other vegetable oils. Roughly 60 % of the brain is made up of lipids, of which an important part is EPA. They are vital for the proper growth and development of the brain and the central nervous system. Essential fatty acids have two major roles. First they are constituents of all cell membranes and in all the tissues in the body; secondly they give rise to highly reactive molecules, the prostaglandins and leukotrienes.

GLA or gamma linolenic acid is very special in its function firstly it helps build healthy cell membranes in every single cell of the body and secondly, GLA converts, inside the body, to a physiologically active substance called prostaglandin E1 (PGE1). GLA and PGE1 together provided by Evening Primrose Oil are the ones what make this oil so useful for restoring the balance of the body system and treating a wide range of disorders.

> The fatty acids are an essential part of nutrition and perform all kinds of vital functions within the body viz.-
> - they give energy
> - they help maintain body temperature
> - they insulate the nerves
> - they cushion and protect tissues
> - they are the part of the structure of every cell in our body and are vital for metabolism.
> - They are precursors of the all important short lived regulating molecules, the Prostaglandins.

Prostaglandins were discovered by a Swedish scientist, Von Euler, in 1930s. He first found these molecules in the seminal fluid and thought they came from prostrate gland, so he called them prostaglandins, later scientists discovered that these molecules were all over the body. Prostaglandins have been found particularly in blood vessel walls, macrophages, platelets, duodenal secretions, nerves and every organ. They have an extremely short life span and most are removed from the blood during single passage through the lungs. They are naturally unstable because they have highly efficient mechanisms which break them down. The very short life span of prostaglandins, make them difficult to administer as drugs, since they have to be given intravenously.

Prostaglandins act as vital cell regulators. They control every cell and every organ in your body on a second- by second basis. The nearest thing to them is hormones, which also have important messenger role.

There are three series of prostaglandins, PG1, PG2, and PG3. Each of these has a different chemical structure and within each series there are different types classified by letters A, B, D, E, F etc. In all, there are at least 50 different prostaglandins and still new ones being discovered.

The three series of prostaglandins are each derived from a different fatty acid. Series 1 and 2 both come from the linoleic acid family. Series 3 is derived from eicosapentaenoic acid, a member of alpha-linolenic acid family and most commonly found in oily sea foods.

Each prostaglandin has a different role to play. Health problems can arise when the different series of prostaglandins are out of balance with each other. The balance between the 1 and 2 series PGs can be influenced by diet. In inflammatory conditions, the end products of arachidonic acid metabolism prostaglandins series 2, cyclo-oxygenase and thromboxane A2- are being produced in too great quantity, whereas PGE 1 is not being produced in enough quantities.

Two of the most widely used drugs- steroids and non- steroidal anti-inflammatory drugs (NSAIDs) work by inhibiting the biosynthesis of prostaglandins. By suppressing the production of prostaglandins the drugs dampen down inflammation. However, the trouble with this drug approach is that all the prostaglandins are knocked out- including the good ones. Evening primrose oil works in a completely different way from these powerful drugs. Instead of stopping the manufacture of prostaglandins, Evening primrose goes on to make the anti-inflammatory prostaglandin E1 hence manipulates the prostaglandins in a natural way.

PROSTAGLANDIN E1 (PGE1) seems to have the most desirable qualities amongst all the prostaglandins and evening primrose oil is most easily converted to prostaglandin E1 . The following is a list of benefits that PGE1 gives to the body-

- It promotes dilation of blood vessels.
- It lowers arterial pressure.
- It inhibits thrombosis.
- It inhibits cholesterol synthesis.
- It inhibits inflammation and controls arthritis.
- It inhibits abnormal cell proliferation.
- It inhibits platelet aggregation.
- It regulates production of saliva and tears.
- It elevates cyclic AMP (adenosine monophosphate)

Due to this Evening Primrose oil is useful on a wide range of symptoms, notable amongst are-

PMS (Pre Menstual Syndrome)-

PMS is a condition which affects the whole system. Six of the most common symptoms experienced by women with PMS are irritability, depression, breast pain, bloating, headaches and clumsiness. However, the cluster of symptoms include swollen ankles, legs, reduced libido, constipation, hot flushes, backache, nausea, acne, cramps, food cravings, lethargy and fatigue on the physical side and on psychological/ emotional side are anxiety, mood swings, suicidal impulses, low self esteem, weeping for no obvious reason, sudden tantrums, lack of concentration and lapses of memory.

PMS can cause havoc to women's lives at worst wrecking relationships, marriages and careers. Evening Primrose oil has been used successfully as part of a treatment program for PMS, since the beginning of 1980's. Trials have consistently proved that most women- more than 80 % of them who suffer from PMS improve on evening primrose oil.

Women suffering from PMS are thought to be low on in essential fatty acids and also considered to be low in the important prostaglandin E1 made from EFAs besides, they also have an imbalance of the various prostaglandins. A shortage of EFAs can lead to an apparent excess of the female hormone prolactin. Prolactin produces changes in mood and fluid metabolism, similar to those found in PMS. It is thought that GLA and PGE1, derived from evening primrose oil, can damp down these effects of prolactin and other hormones.

Though evening primrose oil has an important role to play as nutritional therapy for PMS but other important things are diet, specific minerals and vitamin supplements, exercise, and lifestyle changes to reduce stress. The various vitamins and minerals found useful in controlling PMS are-

- Vitamin C- between 500 mg to 3 g. per day
- B complex tablets appropriate ratio
- Vitamin B6- 50 mg per day
- Zinc- 10 mg a day

However the most suitable dose of evening primrose oil is 1 teaspoon spoon full ie 5 ml per day or minimum of two capsules three times a day after meals. Though ingestion of liquid, may not be palatable to some but a preferable option to avoid the extra gelatin.

FIBROCYSTIC BREAST CONDITION & BREAST PAIN (Mastalgia)

Breast pain, is common in women can be associated with the menstrual cycle. It can occur as part of premenstrual syndrome, in some cases lasting as long as two weeks in every four. Or it may have nothing to do with a woman's menstrual cycle. In such cases the women can have the pain continuously, feeling irritable and depressed, as a result. Typically, the breasts feel heavy and tender, with a lumpy granular sort of texture. Many women usually visit doctors fearing breast cancer.

It is believed that the breast pain is caused by abnormal sensitivity of breast tissue to normal levels of hormones prolactin and oestrogen. Until recently breast pain has been treated with hormone related drugs having their own side effects; however evening primrose oil is an effective alternative with none of the side effects.

There is an interesting relationship between heart disease in men and mastalgia and PMS in women. In societies, where there is a high rate of death from heart disease among young and middle aged men, there is a correspondingly high rate of breast disease and PMS in young and middle aged women.

If a high intake of saturated fat is associated with benign breast disease and other diseases, then increasing the intake of polyunsaturated fatty acids may reverse or prevent the development of mastalgia and PMS. Women with breast disease tend to have high rates of sebum production, which is a marker of EFA deficiency.

A shortage of essential fatty acids in the diet leads to excessive amounts of fibrous tissue. Cysts, which are another common symptom of mastalgia, may form because for some reason the body is making too much of the hormone prolactin, and is short of prostaglandin E1.

Evening primrose oil is useful, as a treatment for breast pain because PGE1 can dampen down the effects of prolactin, may prevent the development of cysts and can help remove lumpiness in the breasts.

Women with breast pain have been found to have normal or near normal levels of linoleic acid. However, they have abnormally low levels of metabolites of linoleic acid. Evening primrose oil works because its active ingredient is GLA, which by passes the metabolic block. So the level of essential fatty acids is brought up to normal.

DIABETES

Even when diabetes is well controlled by insulin and diet, there can still be complications. Diabetes can lead to severe damage to the heart and circulation, to the eyes, to the kidneys and to nerves. The damage to the nerves known medically as diabetic neuropathy- can lead to lots of skin problems, muscles weakness, bladder and intestinal problems and impotence in men. Diabetic neuropathy affects about half of all diabetics and there has been no effective treatment for it.

Another common complication for diabetics is degeneration of the retina of the eye (diabetic retinopathy). This is a common cause of blindness in middle aged people. This happens because diabetes causes swellings in the walls of the arteries feeding the retina and twists in the retinal veins. As a result, there are tiny hemorrhages and the retinal tissue degenerates and dies.

Evening primrose oil is a major breakthrough in the treatment of diabetic neuropathy. It has been found that evening primrose can actually reverse the nerve damage in diabetics. Recent research from scientists from France and Australia has provided evidence that diabetics cannot make GLA normally from linoleic acid in their diet and this inability to make GLA may be a cause of some of the long term complications of diabetes. But GLA given to diabetics with nerve damage can both prevent and reverse diabetic nerve damage.

It has also been found useful to take evening primrose oil to prevent damage to retina. There have been successful trials in Holland where linoleic acid was used, and it was found that the patients with diabetes who took large amounts of linoleic acid stopped the retinas from degenerating. Evening primrose oil works in the same way as linoleic acid, but because it is more powerful, you would not need to take as much. The Dutch researchers have found that the diabetic patients, who are on a diet high in linoleic acid, needed less insulin.

HEART DISEASE, VASCULAR DISORDERS & HIGH BLOOD PRESSURE

Heart disease and diseases of the blood vessels are among the biggest killers, despite a certain amount of controversy over the underlying risk factors which contribute to the coronary deaths, a number are broadly accepted-

- High Cholesterol level in blood
- Platelets that stick together unduly (platelet aggregation)
- High Blood Pressure
- Atheroma clogging up blood vessels
- Vascular spasm

Since 1950s, it has been known that linoleic acid is able to reduce cholesterol levels, but it means taking large quantities of linolenic acid, which would be very high in calories as well as relatively unpalatable. However it has now been realized that the power to reduce cholesterol levels is not so much vested in the linoleic acid itself, but in its metabolites dihomo-gammalinolenic acid (DGLA) and also arachidonic acid.

There is a strong association between the incidence of cardiovascular disease and reduced levels of DGLA. In the metabolic pathway of linoleic acid, DGLA is formed from gamma linolenic acid (GLA), the active ingredient of evening primrose oil. So you need to take only 10 % of evening primrose oil and its 100 times more potent than linoleic acid in reducing cholesterol. Recommended dose is approx 5 mg. per day.

Evening primrose oil has an interesting effect on cholesterol levels. It will only bring down cholesterol levels if they are high, but it will have no effect on cholesterol levels if they are normal or low. This is because evening primrose oil works physiologically to regulate cholesterol metabolism instead of working pharmacologically as a drug.

As the starting cholesterol levels rise, so the relative potency, of the GLA, in evening primrose oil increases. Evening primrose oil is clearly an effective cholesterol lowering agent in those people with plasma cholesterol values above 5mmol/1, in other words, in all but the lowest 20 % of cholesterol levels.

Like other PUFAs, evening primrose oil either has no effect on HDL (high density lipoprotein) cholesterol or actually increases it. The cholesterol-lowering action of evening primrose oil is entirely because it is able to lower LDL (low density lipoprotein) cholesterol. It is the LDL cholesterol which is harmful and which needs to be lowered in order to reduce the risk of heart attack. HDL cholesterol is desirable because it actually helps to transport cholesterol away from places where it may be harmful. Evening primrose oil has the very beneficial effect of raising the HDL / LDL ratio.

A risk factor for cardiovascular disorders occurs when the platelets in the blood aggregate abnormally- they bunch up and stick together. Evening primrose oil is very effective in stopping this process.

The clotting agents in the blood are called platelets. When platelets stick to cholesterol deposits this quickly leads to a clot, which can block the flow of blood. When a blood clot forms in an artery or a vein it is called a thrombosis. This blocks the circulation in the area. A clot in a coronary artery is a coronary thrombosis. In brain it's a stroke. Evening primrose oil helps, because the GLA in evening primrose oil easily converts to DGLA, which is known to be able to reduce platelet aggregation. Besides, evening primrose oil coverts to prostaglandin E1 and PGE 1 is one of the most potent known inhibitors of platelet aggregation.

People with high blood pressure run a greater risk of experiencing arteriosclerosis, heart failure, stroke, and kidney disease. Evening primrose oil has been considered more effective in lowering blood pressure than much higher doses of other polyunsaturated fatty acids. Diets rich in polyunsaturated fatty acids may not only arrest the progression of atheroma, but may actually reverse it, allowing the obstruction to be cleared. Taking evening primrose oil as supplement would be worthwhile even for those people whose cardiovascular system is already damaged.

CANCER

A research in South Africa (published in South African Medical Journal) showed that gammalinolenic acid, taken from evening primrose oil, reduced cancer cell growth up to 70%. Six different laboratories in four different countries have now obtained similar results that polyunsaturated fatty acids normalize human cancer cells, the tests had been conducted on at least nine different human malignant cell lines, including cancers of the liver, bone, esophagus, breast, prostrate and skin. In all these tests, the normal cells remain unaffected.

What researchers observed that GLA in evening primrose oil may be working in three different ways-

1. Lipid peroxides- When human cancer cells are exposed to polyunsaturated fatty acids in the laboratory, the cells generate large amounts of substances called lipid peroxides and die. Several PUFAs have been tried and GLA seems to be the best PUFA- it highly toxic to malignant cells, but has no toxic effects whatsoever on the normal cells.

2. It by-passes the delta-6-desaturase enzyme block. Cancer is a known blocking agent of the metabolic pathway of linoleic acid. This block occurs at the first step, between linoleic acid and gammalinolenic acid, by inhibiting the delta-6-desaturase enzyme. GLA in evening primrose oil by-passes this block by starting at the second stage in the metabolic pathway. This means that GLAQ can convert to DGLA and then to prostaglandin E1 without hindrance.

3. Prostaglandins- Another way in which polyunsaturated fatty acids might be controlling cancer cells is by being converted into prostaglandins. Prostaglandins derived from PUFAs may inhibit the proliferation of human and animal tumour cells, and reversed transformed cells.

The aim of using evening primrose oil in the treatment of cancer cells from proliferating, without affecting healthy cells, which is different from the orthodox treatment using chemotherapy or radiation which is toxic to cancerous as well as healthy cells, with unpleasant side effect. Since the findings of evening primrose oil are mostly subjective and not conclusive, some therapists may have their doubts. However, evening primrose oil works more at physiological level as a nutritional supplement without any side effect, should be good reason to use it, as it will also help controlling side effects of orthodox treatments like chemotherapy and radiation.

AIDS, Viral Infections and post viral fatigue Syndrome

The most exciting development with evening primrose oil in recent years is its effect on viral infections. This could herald a radically new low risk approach to treating viral infections, including AIDS. Essential fatty acids are particularly important because they have direct virus killing effects and are lethal at surprisingly low concentrations to many viruses. They are also required for the anti viral actions of the body's own natural virus fighter, interferon.

But in order to effective as an antiviral agent, interferon needs prostaglandins, which are converted from essential fatty acids. Without the EFAs the prostaglandins, the antiviral actions of interferon are lost or certainly much diminished.

It is now known that essential fatty acids are severely depleted with AIDS and reduced in patients with glandular fever and other viral infections. This may be caused by the effects of the virus itself, rather than any lack of essential fatty acids in the diet. The rationale, for giving evening primrose oil, is to increase the supply of the metabolites of the parent EFAs so that the EFAs can do their viral killing work and also help interferon do its virus fighting job.

ECZEMA

As long ago as the 1930s it was known that essential fatty acids are vital for healthy skin and hair. But it is only in the last decade people realized the efficacy of evening primrose oil on skin disorders specially eczema. In studies it has been found that whenever there are low levels of essential fatty acids-

* The skin becomes scaly, rough and sheds dandruff-like scales. In severe deficiency, an eczema like dermatitis may develop and the skin may break down.

* Wounds take longer to heal

* There is greater water loss from the skin, making it drier and making it age more quickly.

Atopic eczema is chronic, patchy, mild inflammation of the surface of the skin, which almost always begins in infancy or early childhood. It can be made worse by irritants, but often occurs without any apparent cause. In recent years evening primrose oil had excellent result in the treatment of atopic eczema, in both adults and children.

All studies done so far agree that people with atopic eczema have below normal levels of GLA , DGLA, AA, PGE1 and metabolites of alpha linolenic acid. The enzyme delta-6-desaturase is needed to get from linoleic acid to the next step and from alpha-linolenic acid to the next step.

The evening primrose oil completely by-passes this enzyme block by starting at the next stage in the metabolic pathway of the linoleic acid family. Please note that the improvement does not happen overnight as it take four to 12 weeks after starting ingestion of evening primrose oil.

ASTHMA, HAY FEVER ALLERGIES AND OTHER ATOPIC CONDITIONS

On the face of it, eczema, asthma, hay fever and allergies all sound like very different conditions but in fact a lot in common- they are all to do with abnormal body defense mechanism called Atopy. Atopy or a generalized allergic response can show itself as any or all of a variety of conditions.

Atopic eczema is closely linked with other atopic conditions like asthma and hay fever, and it is also common to find other members of the family suffering from these conditions. It has been a common knowledge that people with eczema, asthma and allergies have something wrong with their immune system mainly due to fatty acids abnormality which affects various other parts regulating the immune system particularly PGE1 and T lymphocytes.

Evening primrose oil helps to correct the faulty immune system in people with atopic conditions, which is because it converts to PGE1 , which stimulates the T- lymphocytes playing an all important role in the immune system.

HYPERACTIVE CHILDREN

It seems evening primrose oil works especially well on atopic children having family history of such ailments as eczema, asthma, allergies, hay fever or migraine. The mothers of hyperactive children are often found to have migraine or may suffer from pre menstrual tension or post natal depression. Evening primrose oil has helped to improve dramatically the lives of countless children and their families. When combined with nutritional and dietary approach evening primrose oil work wonders on hyperactive children. The key things to take out of the child's diet are artificial coloring, flavoring and preservatives.

Hyperactive children might be deficient in PGE1, which helps control the immune system and has an influence on such things like asthma, behaviour and thirst (via the kidneys) Salicylates, in aspirin and even in seemingly innocent foods as apples, oranges, peaches, strawberries, grapes, cherries, almonds and cucumbers also are known to block the formation of prostaglandins, therefore should be excluded from the diet. Parents are advised to give children only fresh foods and avoid anything with vit. E additions, however other vitamins and mineral supplements are very helpful. Since hyperactive children are are found to be very low in zinc and magnesium. So the evening primrose oil should be taken with its cofactors, which are zinc, vitamin B6, nicotinamide (vitamin B3) and vitamin C.

RHEUMATOID ARTHRITIS

Rheumatoid arthritis is the inflammatory form of arthritis, a chronic condition affecting connective tissues, mainly of joints and can be very painful. Recent studies using evening primrose oil and evening primrose oil along with fish oil has provided substantial improvement in their conditions and helped them reduce or give up treatment with conventional anti inflammatory drugs. However, as yet there is no evidence that they act as agents which actually modify the disease.

SKIN, HAIR, EYES, NAILS & BUST

The two major essential fatty acids, linoleic acid and gamma linolenic acid, in which evening primrose oil is rich, are natural skin nutrients. Linoleic acid and gamma linolenic acid are vital components of the structure of all cell membranes and are normally converted by the body into prostaglandins. Prostaglandins play an important role in maintaining skin health.

When evening primrose oil is applied directly to the skin, linoleic acid and gamma linolenic acid have a profound effect on reducing trans-epidermal water loss, therefore acting as a natural moisturizer and help slow down the aging process.

The discovery that evening primrose oil can cure brittle nails was by chance. A medical trial was being conducted, in Scotland, using evening primrose oil for two conditions which make the eyes and mouth dry and painful (Sjogren's syndrome and Sicca syndrome). It was found that not only did their dry eyes and mouths get better, but their brittle nails dramatically improved at the same time.

An unforeseen side effect of evening primrose oil in some women, consuming evening primrose oil since a long time, is increased bust size; however they noticed that they have not put on weight anywhere else in the body.

It has been observed that animals deprived of essential fatty acids suffered loss of their fur as well as dandruff like conditions. Use of evening primrose oil has improved chronic dandruff and controlled hair loss.

Side Effects

Though there are no noticeable side effects of evening primrose oil, being used in capsule form or ingested directly as liquid, but there are reports of seizures with the use of evening primrose oil. People at risk of seizures should avoid using it. Evening primrose oil lowers blood pressure in animals, but effects in humans are not clear. Headache, stomach pain, nausea and loose stools may occur.

Recommendation

It is recommended to consume one tea spoon (5 ml.) cold pressed evening primrose oil, preferably from known source (manufacturer or repacker) and under guidance of a therapist or practitioner. At FM's Aromatherapy, we repack our Evening Primrose after ensuring the quality and percentage of GLA available in the oil, no synthetic preservatives or flavoring agents are added. **The oil is available through mail order contact fmsaroma@yahoo.co.uk, aromatantra@yahoo.com.**

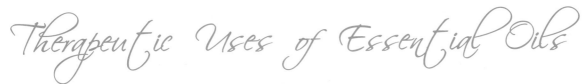

Therapeutic Uses of Essential Oils

(READY - REFERENCE)

For therapeutic effects of essential Oils-

The following list has been compiled from some of the most reliable references available, plus the author's own experience. **Bold type** are the ones which are commonly used in connection with the particular ailment.

ABDOMINAL CRAMP	Aniseed; Basil; Bergamot; **Caraway**; Chamommile, Clove bud; **Fennel;** Lavender, **Marjoram**, sweet; Melissa, true; **Nutmeg**; Orange, bitter.
ABSCESSES BOILS	Cajuput; **German** Chamomile; Clove bud; Lavender; Lemon; Niaouli; **Palmarosa, Tea tree** (infection); Thyme red (infection); Thyme, sweet.
ACNE	Bergamot; Cajuput; Cedarwood; **German** Chamomile; **Geranium; Juniper** berry; **Lavender**; Lemon; Neroli; Palmarosa, Patchouli; Petitgrain; Rosemary; Sandalwood; **Tea tree**
AIR DISINFECTANT	**Basil, Citronella, Eucalyptus;** Grapefruit; Lemon; **Lemon grass**; Melissa, **Pine; Rosemary**, Sage; Thyme
ALLERGIES/ SENSITIVE SKIN	**German Chamomile;** Clary sage; Neroli; Hyssop; **Lavender**; Patchouli; Sandalwood
ANTI-AGEING	**Carrot**, Clary sage; **Frankincense; Geranium; Lavender;** Marjoram (sweet); Neroli; Orange (bitter); Palmarosa, Patchouli; Rose Otto; **Sandalwood;** Vertiver; Ylang Ylang
ANXIETY	**Basil;** Bergamot; Cedarwood; **Roman Chamomile; Clary sage; Geranium; Helichrysm, Lavender;** Lemon; Marjoram (sweet); Melissa ; Neroli; Orange (sweet); Patchouli; Petitgrain; **Rose Otto; Rosemary, Rosewood; Sandalwood;** Thyme; Vertiver; Ylang Ylang
LACK OF APPETITE	Bergamot; **Dill seed,** Roman Chamomile; **Coriander; Fennel;** Mandarin, **Oregano.**
ARTHRITIS	**Basil, Black pepper; Cajuput; Clove,** German Chamomile; Coriander; Cypress; Eucalyptus; **Juniper;** Lavandin; **Lavender;** Marjoram (sweet); Niaouli; Rosemary, Sage; Savory; Thyme (sweet), **Wintergreen**
ASTHMA	Aniseed; **Basil,** Bergamot; Cajuput; Cedarwood; Roman Chamomile; **Eucalyptus; Frankincense;** Hyssop; Lavender; Lemon; Mandarin; Marjoram; Neroli; Niaouli; Pine; Peppermint; Rose Otto; **Rosemary; Sage;** Thyme (sweet), **Evening Primrose Oil (Oral).**

BAD BREATH	Basil; Bergamot; Caraway; **Fennel seed,** Grapefruit; **Lemon;** Myrrh; Nutmeg; Orange (bitter); **Peppermint; Spearmint,** Thyme (sweet)
BED WETTING	**Cypress; Mandarin, Orange,** Pine, Rosemary
BRONCHITIS	Aniseed; Basil; Bay; **Black pepper;** Cajuput; Cedarwood; Clove bud; Cypress; **Eucalyptus;** Frankincense; **Ginger;** Hyssop; Juniper; Lavender; Lemon; sweet Marjoram; Myrrh; Niaouli; Pine; Rose Otto; Rosemary; Sage; Sandalwood; Tea tree; **Thyme red;** Thyme (sweet)
BRUISES	Camphor; **German Chamomile;** Fennel; Hyssop; Helichrysm, **Lavender;** Lemon; Marjoram (sweet); Myrrh; Rosemary; Sage
BURNS	Banzoin; **German Chamomile;** Geranium; Helichrysm, **Lavender; Palmarosa,** Rosewood, Sage; Tea tree
CANDIDA (THRUSH)	Bergamot; Cinnamon bark; Eucalyptus; **Geranium;** Oregano, Rose Otto; Rosemary; Sage; **Tea tree;** Thyme (sweet)
CATARRH	**Basil,** Benzoin; **Black pepper; Cajuput;** Cedarwood; **Eucalyptus,** Lavender; Lemon; Marjoram; Myrrh; Niaouli; Peppermint; Rosemary; Sage; Sandalwood; Tagetes; Tea tree
CELLULITE	Black Pepper; Cedarwood; Cinnamon, **Cypress; Fennel;** Geranium; **Grapefruit, Juniper Berry,** Lavender, **Lemongrass, Melissa,** Patchouli; Rosemary; Sage; Sandalwood
CIRRHOSIS	Clary sage; Juniper; Helichrysm, Lavender, Rosemary
CONSTIPATION	**Aniseed,** Basil; Black Pepper; Roman Chamomile; **Coriander; Dill, Fennel;** Ginger; Juniper; Mandarin; bitter Orange; Rosemary
COUGHS AND COLDS	**Basil;** Bay; **Black pepper;** Cedarwood; Clove, Eucalyptus; Geranium; Ginger, Juniper; Lavender; Lemon; Marjoram; Peppermint; Pine; Tea tree; Thyme sweet
CRAMP	Basil; Cajuput; **Roman Chamomile;** Cypress; **Eucalyptus, Lavender;** Mandarin; Marjoram, sweet; Rosemary; Valerian
CUTS / WOUNDS	Benzoin; Bergamot; Camphor; Cedarwood; **German Chamomile;** Clove bud; Cypress; Eucalyptus; Frankincense; Geranium; Hyssop; **Lavender;** Lemon; Myrrh; Niaouli; Orange bitter; Palmarosa, Rose Otto; Rosemary; Sage; **Tea tree**
CYSTITIS	Basil sweet; Bergamot; Cajuput; German Chamomile; Clove bud; Coriander; Eucalyptus; **Geranium,** Hyssop; **Juniper; Lavender,** Niaouli; Peppermint; **Sandalwood;** Thyme red; Thyme, sweet.
DEBILITY	**Basil;** Camphor; Cinnamon bark; Clove bud; Coriander; **Geranium;** Hyssop; **Lavandin;** Marjoram sweet; Peppermint; Pine; **Rosewood;** Savory; Tea tree; Thyme, red; **Thyme, sweet;** Valerian.

DEPRESSION	**Basil;** Bergamot; Chamomile; Cinnamon bark; Cypress; **Geranium;** Grapefruit, Hyssop; Juniper; **Jasmine,** Lemon grass; **Melissa, Neroli;** Niaouli; Orange; Petitgrain; Pine; Rosemary; Rose Otto; Rosewood; Ylang Ylang; Evening Primrose Oil (Oral)
DERMATITIS	**Benzoin; Cade,** Cajuput; **German Chamomile;** Moroccan Chamomile; Eucalyptus; Geranium; Hyssop; **Juniper;** Lemon, Lavender; Palmarosa, **Patchouli;** Rose Otto; Sage; **Tea Tree,** Thyme (sweet), **Evening Primrose Oil (Oral),** Cinnamon.
DIABETES	Clary Sage; Evening Primrose Oil (Oral), Eucalyptus; Geranium; Juniper; Lemon; Pine; Rosemary, Thyme (sweet); Vertiver
DIARRHOEA	Basil, Black pepper; Chamomile; **Coriander, Cinnamon bark;** Clove bud; Geranium; Ginger; **Juniper;** Lemon; Marjoram (sweet); Myrrh; Niaouli; Nutmeg; Peppermint; **Tea Tree,** Sandalwood; Savory
EAR ACHE	Basil; Cajuput; Roman Chamomile; **Lavender;** Rosemary; **Tea tree**
ECZEMA	Basil; **Benzoin;** Cajuput; German Chamomile; Moroccan Chamomile; Clove bud; Eucalyptus; **Frankincense;** Geranium; Hyssop; **Juniper;** Lavender; **Myrrh; Niaouli;** Patchauli; Rose Otto; Sandalwood; **Tea tree,** Thyme (sweet), Evening Primrose Oil (Oral).
EPILEPSY	Basil; Cajuput; **Clary sage; Lavender; Marjoram (sweet); parsley leaf;** Rosemary; Thyme (sweet)
FLATULENCE	Angelica, **Aniseed;** Basil; Bergamot; Black pepper; **Caraway; Coriander;** Fennel; Ginger; Lavender; Mandarin; Marjoram (sweet); Niaouli; Orange (bitter); Peppermint; Thyme (sweet)
FLU	Basil, **Cajuput;** Clove bud; Coriander; **Eucalyptus;** Lavender; **Lemon; Lemongrass;** Myrrh; Niaouli; Peppermint; Pine; **Rosemary;** Sage; **Tea tree;** Thyme (sweet)
FLUID RETENTION	Cedarwood; **Cypress;** Fennel; Geranium; **Grapefruit, Juniper berry;** Lemon; Orange; Pine; **Rosemary**
FRIGIDITY	Aniseed, **Black pepper;** Clove, Clary sage, Moroccan Chamomile; Frankincense; **Ginger; Jasmine;** Neroli,; Rose Otto; **Sandalwood; Ylang Ylang**
FUNGAL INFECTIONS (SKIN)	Cypress; **Geranium;** Lavender; Niaouli; **Oregano,** Patchouli; Pine; Rosemary; Sage; Sandalwood; Savory; Tagetes; **Tea tree;** Thyme (sweet)
GASTRIC ULCERS	Basil; **German Chamomile;** Fennel; Geranium; Lemon;Lavender, Marjoram (sweet); Niaouli, **Oregano, Tea Tree,**
GASTRO ENTERITIS	Basil, Bergamot; Cajuput; Caraway; **German Chamomile;** Moroccan Chamomile; Clove bud; **Coriander;** Cypress; Fennel; Juniper berry; Lavender; Lemongrass; Mandarin (sweet); Niaouli; Nutmeg; Patchouli; Peppermint; Sage; **Tea tree;** Thyme
GINGIVITIS	Clary sage; **Cypress,** Eucalyptus, Juniper; **Lemon;** Sage, Tea Tree.
GLANDULAR INFLAMMATION	Clary Sage; Geranium; Pine; Rosemary Sage; Thyme (sweet)

GOUT	Basil; Cajuput, Eucalyptus, Roman Chamomile; Fennel; Juniper; Lavender, Lemon; Pine; Rosemary
GUM INFECTIONS (PYORRHOEA)	Cinnamon bark; Clove bud; **Cypress;** Geranium; Lavender, Juniper; Peppermint, Rosemary; **Tea tree**
HAEMORRHOIDS	Bergamot; Cajuput; Clary Sage; Cypress; **Frankincense;** Geranium; **Myrrh;** Neroli; Niaouli; **Patchouli;** Sandalwood; **Tea tree;** Valerian
HEADACHE	**Basil;** Roman Chamomile; Eucalyptus; Lavender; Lemon; Marjoram (sweet); Melissa (true); Peppermint; Rosemary
HEARTBURN	Moroccan Chamomile; Roman Chamomile; Peppermint; Sandalwood
HEPATITIS	Basil; Clove bud; Eucalyptus; Juniper; Lemongrass; Myrrh; Niaouli; Petitgrain; Rosemary
HERPES	Nia6uli (genital); Sage. Bergamot; Eucalyptus; Geraniu m; Lavender; Lemon; Niaouli; Sage
HICCUPS	Basil, Mandarin, Tangerine.
HIGH BLOOD PRESSURE	Basil, sweet, Clary sage, Juniper; Lavender; Lemon; Marjoram (sweet); Ylang Ylang
HYSTERIA	Lemongrass; Helichrysm, Melissa (true)
IMPOTENCE	Aniseed; Black Pepper; Cinnamon bark; Ginger; Peppermint; Pine; Rose Otto; Savory; Thyme (sweet); Ylang Ylang
INDIGESTION	Aniseed; Basil; Bergamot; **Black Pepper;** Caraway; Coriander; **Dill; Fennel; Ginger;** Lemon; Lemongrass; Mandarin; Melissa, true; Orange (bitter); Orange, sweet; **Peppermint;** Rosemary.
INFLAMMATION	**Chamomile(German);** Clary sage; Frankincense; Geranium; **Lavender;** Myrrh; Peppermint; **Petitgrain;** Rose Otto; Sandalwood
INSECT BITES	Basil; **Cajuput; Lavender;** Melissa, true; Niaouli; Sage; **Tea tree;** Thyme (sweet)
INSECT REPELLENT	**Basil;** Cedarwood; **Citronella;** Clove bud; Eucalyptus; Geranium; Lemon; Lemongrass; Peppermint; **Thyme**
INSOMNIA	Bergamot; Chamomile, Roman; **Clary Sage;** Cypress; Geranium; **Lavender;** Mandarin; **Marjoram (Sweet)** Melissa true; Neroli; bitter Orange; sweet Orange; Rose Otto; **Sandalwood;** Valerian; Ylang Ylang
IRRITATION (SKIN)	**German Chamomile;** Cedarwood; **Lavender;** Neroli; Peppermint; **Sandalwood**
KIDNEY, GENERAL	Cedarwood; Eucalyptus, Fennel; Geranium; **Juniper;** Lavender; Lemon; Niaouli; Pine; Sage; Sandalwood; Thyme (red); Thyme (sweet)
KIDNEY INFECTIONS	Clove bud; Coriander; Myrrh; Sandalwood; Sage Savory; Thyme
KIDNEY STONES	Fennel; Geranium; Hyssop; **Juniper;** Lemon.

LABOUR PAIN	Clary, Sage; Fennel; Nutmeg
LARYNGITIS	Black Pepper; Cajuput; Cypress; Eucalyptus; **Lemon;** Myrrh; Niaouli; Peppermint; Sage; Sandalwood
LIVER SLUGGISH	Basil; Black Pepper; Cajuput; Moroccan Chamomile; Juniper; **Lemon;** Lemongrass; Melissa true; Peppermint; Rosemary; Thyme (sweet); Vertiver
LOW BLOOD PRESSURE	**Black Pepper, Cinnamon;** Clove bud; Hyssop, Lemon, Neroli; Peppermint; **Rosemary; Sage;** Savory; Thyme, (Sweet)
LUMBAGO	Aniseed; **Eucalyptus;** Fennel; Geranium; Lavender, Sandalwood
MENOPAUSE	Aniseed; Basil; Bergamot; Roman Chamomile; **Clary Sage,** Cypress; Fennel; Geranium; Hyssop; Jasmine; Juniper; **Lavender;** Lemon; Mandarin; Melissa (true); Peppermint; Pine; **Rose Otto;** Rosemary; Sage; **Sandalwood,** Evening Primrose Oil (Oral).
MENTAL FATIGUE	**Basil;** Cajuput; Clove bud; Coriander; Juniper berry; Lavender; Neroli; Peppermint; Rosemary; Rosewood
MIGRAINE	Aniseed; Basil; German Chamomile; **Eucalyptus, Lavender;** Marjoram (sweet); Melissa (true); Neroli; **Peppermint; Rosemary**
LACK OF MILK	(BREAST FEEDING) Aniseed; Dill; **Fennel**
MOUTH ULCERS	Basil, Clove bud; Geranium; **Juniper;** Lemon; Myrrh; Niaouli; Rose Otto; Sage; Sandalwood, **Tea tree**
MUSCULAR PAIN	Bergamot; Black Pepper; Camphor; **Cajuput;** Cinnamon; German; Chamomile; Moroccan Chamomile; Roman Chamomile; Eucalyptus; Frankincense; Juniper; Lavender, Nutmeg; Rosemary; Thyme (sweet); Vertiver
NAUSEA	Black Pepper; Caraway; Fennel; Ginger; Mandarin; Melissa, true; **Peppermint;** Sandalwood, **Spearmint.**
NERVOUS EXHAUSTION	**Basil;** Clary Sage; Clove bud; Coriander; **Geranium;** Helichrysm, Lavender; Savory; Tea tree; Thyme (sweet)
NEURALGIA	Camphor; Roman Chamomile; Clove bud; Eucalyptus; Ginger; Helichrysm, Juniper; **Lavender;** Marjoram, sweet, Peppermint; Pine; Rosemary; Sandalwood
NEURITIS	**German Chamomile; Roman Chamomile;** Clary; Sage; Cypress; Clove; Juniper; Lavender, Niaouli; Thyme (sweet)
OEDEMA	Cedarwood; **Cypress;** Eucalyptus, Geranium; Ginger, **Juniper;** Berry, Orange; Patchouli; **Rosemary;** Sage; Sandalwood.
OSTEOPOROSIS	Eucalyptus; Lavender; Lemon; Lemongrass; Rosemary; Sage OVARIES Clary; Cypress; Rosemary; Sage; Ylang Ylang, Evening Primrose Oil (Oral)
PALPITATIONS	Aniseed; Fennel; Geranium, **Lavender;** Mandarin; Melissa (true); Neroli; Petitgrain; Rose, Rosemary; Valerian; Ylang Ylang

LACK OF PERIODS	Aniseed; Roman Chamomile; Cinnamon bark; **Clary Sage;** Fennel; **Juniper,** berry; Peppermint Rosemary; Sage; Tagetes; Thyme sweet; Veltiver, Evening Primrose Oil (Oral)
PAINFUL PERIODS	Aniseed; Basil (congestion); Chamomile, German (congestion); **ClarySage,** Cypress (congestion); Fennel **Geranium (congestion);** Juniper; Lavender Marjoram, sweet Peppermint; Pine; Sage (congestion), Evening Primrose Oil (Oral).
SCANTY PERIODS	Basil, Chamomile, Roman; Clary Sage (hormonal); Fennel; **Juniper;** Berry, Lavender; Melissa, true (hormonal); Rosemary; **Rose Otto** (hormonal); Thyme sweet, Veltiver.
PERSPIRATION	Basil; **Cypress;** Geranium; Lavender; Neroli; **Pine,** Sage, Evening Primrose Oral.
PREMENSTRUAL SYNDROME (PMS)	Bergamot, **Chamomile,** Roman; **Clary Sage; Geranium;** Lavender; Melissa, true, **Rose Otto;** Neroli; Sage (congestion); Sandalwood, Veltiver
PROSTRATE (Enlarged)	Basil; Caraway; Cypress.
PSORIASIS	**Benzoin;** Bergamot; **Cade,** Cajuput; Chamomile German; **Juniper berry,** Lavender; Lemon, Niaouli; Patchauli, **Myrrh,** Sandalwood, Peppermint.
RESPIRATORY INFECTION	**Frankincense;** Lemon; Niaouli; Peppermint, Petitgrain; Pine; Rosewood; Tagetes; Tea Tree, **Thyme red.**
RHEUMATISM	Bay, Basil; **Black Pepper;** Cajuput; Camphor; Clove bud; **Eucalyptus;** Frankincense; Geranium (inflammation); **Ginger** (warming); Hyssop; Juniper; Lavandin; **Lavender;** Lemongrass; Marjoram, sweet; Myrrh; Niaouli; **Nutmeg** (analgesic); Petitgrain (nervous); Pine; **Rosemary** (stiffness); Sage; Savory; Thyme, sweet (tonic), **Winter green.**
SCARS	Cedarwood-, Frankincense; Geranuim, Hyssop; Lavender; Myrrh; Patchouli.
SCIATICA	**Camphor; Chamomile,** Roman; Clove bud; **Eucalyptus; Ginger;** Juniper berry; Lavandin; Marjoram, sweet; Peppermint; Pine; Rosemary; Sandalwood
SHINGLES	Clove bud; Eucalyptus; Frankincense; Geranium; **German Chamomile, Lavender,** Marjoram, Niaouli; Peppermint; Sage; **Tea Tree,** Thyme, sweet
SHOCK	**Chamomile, Roman; Helichrysm, Mandarin;** Melissa, true; Neroli; Peppermint; Ylang ylang
SINUSITIS	Bay, Basil, **Cajuput;** Clove bud; **Eucalyptus;** Hyssop; Marjoram, Niaouli; **Peppermint;** Pine; **Rosemary; Sage;** Tea tree; Thyme, sweet
CRACKED / CHAPPED SKIN	**Benzoin,** Chamamile, German, **Patchauli,** Rose Otto; **Sandalwood**
DRY SKIN	Chamomile, German; Chamomile, Roman; Geranium; Lavender; Neroli; Petitgrain; **Rose Otto; Sandalwood; Vertiver**
MATURE SKIN	Benzoin; **Clary Sage;** Fennel; **Frankincense; Geranium, Lavender;** Myrrh; Neroli; **Rose, Sandalwood.**

OILY SKIN (With OPEN PORES)	Cedarwood; Cypress, **Frankincense, Geranium, Juniper Berry,** Lemon. Lavender; Petitgrain; Rose mar Ylang ylang.
SENSITIVE SKIN	**Chamomile,** German; Geranium; Neroli; **Rose Otto; Sandalwood.**
SORE THROAT	Bergamot; Clove bud; Eucalyptus; **Geranium** (inflammation); Lavender (inflammation); Lemon; Lemongrass, Myrrh, Peppermint; Pine; Niaouli; **Sandalwood** (soothing); Thyme
SPRAINS	Fennel; Chamomile, German; Hyssop, **Lavender; Marjoram,** sweet; Nutmeg (analgesic); **Rosemary**
STIMULANT	**Basil;** Cypress; **Malissa,** Marjoram sweet; Niaouli, **Rosemary**
STRETCH MARKS	Carrot Seed; Cedarwood, **Frankincense; Geranium; Lavender;** Myrrh;
SUNBURN	**Chamomile G,** Geranium; **Lavender;** Sandalwood
SWEATY SMELLS	**Cypress;** Ginger, Nutmeg; **Pine;** Sage; Savory; Thyme, red; Thyme, sweet
TENDONITIS	**Chamomile German; Chamomile Roman;** Frankincense; Juniper berry; **Lavender,** Pine; **Rosemary**
THREAD VEINS	Chamomile, German; **Chamomile, Roman;** Cypress; Frankincense; **Lavender;** Lemon; Neroli; Orange, sweet; Patchouli; Peppermint; **Rose Otto**
OVERACTIVE THYROID	**Clary sage,** Clove bud; Marjoram, sweet, Myrrh + **Evening Primrose Oil (Oral)**
TONIC (CIRCULATION)	Cedarwood (lymph); Cypress; **Black Pepper, Ginger, Rosemary** (blood); Sage; Sandalwood; Thyme, sweet
TONIC (MUSCLES)	**Black Pepper;** Cinnamon; **Ginger, Lavender**
TONSILLITIS	Clove bud; Eucalyptus; Geranium; Lemon; Niaouli; Rosemary; Sage; **Sandalwood, Tea Tree,** Thyme, sweet
TOOTHACHE	Black Pepper; Cajuput; Chamomile, Roman (teething); **Clove bud;** Ginger; Nutmeg; Pine; Sage, **Tea Tree.**
TRAVEL SICKNESS	Caraway; Ginger; Helichrysm, **Peppermint, Spearmint**
ULCERS	Benzoin; **Chamomile German; Geranium; Lavender;** Lemon; Myrrh, **Tea Tree**
URINARY TRACT INFECTIONS	Bergamot, Chamomile, Eucalyptus, Frankincense, Geranium, **Juniper, Lavender, Palmarosa, Sandalwood, Tea tree,** Thyme.
VAGINITIS	Chamomile, German; Clary Sage; Lavender; **Niaouli (infection); Tea tree (infection); Thyme red (infection);** Thyme, sweet
VARICOSE ULCERS	Benzoin; Chamomile G.; **Cypress, Geranium; Lavender;** Lemon; Niaouli
VARICOSE VEINS	Basil; Cajuput; Clary, Sage, **Cypress; Juniper (stimulant);** Lemon; Neroli; Niaouli; **Patchouli (decongestant);** Peppermint (cooling); Rosemary (astringent); Sandalwood (soothing); Tea tree; Valerian
VERRUCAE	Lemon; **Oregano, Tea Tree,** Thyme sweet.
VERTIGO	Basil, **Caraway;** Lavender; Lemon; **Helichrysm,** Marjoram, sweet; Melissa, true; Orange; bitter
WRINKLES	Frankincense; Geranium, **Lavender,** Palmarosa, **Rose Otto, Sandalwood.**

Glossary of Names

Abortifacient	Agent which can cause a miscarriage.
Amenorrhea	Abnormal absence of menstruation.
Anti – Allergic	Preventing Allergies.
Aromatology	The Study of essential oils for health.
Astringent	Contracting bodily tissues.
Balsamic	Soothing, Restorative Properties.
Carminative	Relieving flatulence (wind).
Chemotype	Plant grown from cutting in order to propagate plant with known chemical constituent.
Chemovar	Another name for chemotype (var = variety).
Cholagogue	Stimulating flow of bile.
Cicatrisant	Healing, promoting scar tissue formation.
Cohobation	Water used for distillation re-directed into system, to be used repeatedly in a closed cycle.
Cytophylactic	Encouraging cell regeneration.
Diuretic	Stimulating the secretion of urine.
Dysmenorrhea	Abnormally painful or difficult menstruation.
Emmenagogue	Inducing menstruation.
Emulsion	A fluid formed by the suspension of one liquid in another, e.g. oil and water.
Endothelium	The tissues covering the inside surfaces of the body.
Epithelium	The tissues covering the outside surfaces of the body.
Expectorant	Aids removal of catarrh.
Fixed oil	Non - volatile lubricating extract from seeds or nuts, e.g. sunflower oil or almond oil.
Galactogogue	Bringing on the flow of milk.
Hepatic	Tonic to the liver.

Hypatoxic	Toxic to the liver.
Hypertension	High blood pressure.
Hypertensive	That which raises blood pressure.
Hypotension	Low blood pressure.
Hypotensive	Lowers blood pressure.
Hormonal	Balances (or regulates) the body's hormone secretion.
Immuno-stimulant	Stimulating the body's own natural defense system.
Lipolytic	Breaks down fat.
Mucolytic	Breaks down mucus.
Nervine	Nerve tonic.
Neurotoxic	Toxic to the nervous system.
Osmology	The study of smell.
Phytotherapy	Use of the whole plant, as well as the essential oil, to aid healing.
Probiotic	That which favors the beneficial bacteria in the body, while inhibiting harmful microbes. Literally 'favouring life' as opposed to anti-biotic, 'hostile to life'.
Psycho-neuro-immunology	The study of the inter - relationship and mental effects of the mind, nervous system and body's defense system.
Purgative	Causes evacuation of the bowels.
Quencher	Quenches; i.e. suppresses unwanted possible secondary effects.
Rube-facient	Increases local circulation, making skin red.
Scarification	Making a series of small cuts - a method of extracting essence from citrus fruit peel.
Sedative	Producing a calming effect.
Spasmolytic	Relieving muscle spasm or cramp.
Stimulant	Having a rousing, uplifting effect on body and mind.
Stomachic	Good for stomach.
Sudorific	Inducing perspiration.
Synergy	Literally means 'working together'; the phenomenon that occurs when two or more substances used together give a more effective result than any one of the substances used alone.
Vaso-constrictive	Causes contraction of the blood vessels.
Vulnerary	Healing agent for cuts, wounds and sores.

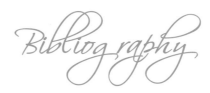

Bibliography

(Author / Title / Publishers)

1. Shirley Price - Aromatherapy workbook- Thomsans (1993), 77-85, Fulham Palace Road, Hammersmith, London.

2. Daniele Ryman - Aromatherapy - Bantan Books (Feb. 1993 1540, Broad- way, New York.

3. Stephaine Tourles - The Herbal Body Book - Storey Publishing (Feb. 1995), Storey Comm. Inc. School House Road, Pownel Vermont.

4. Shirley Price - Aromatherapy for Common Ailments - Simon & Schuster Inc. (1991), Rockfeller Centre, 1230 Avenue of Americas, New York.

5. Ernest Guenther - The Essential oils (vol. 1-6), van Nostrand co. (1982) Robert E. Krieger Pub. Co. Inc., Malabar, Florida.

6. Richard J. Wagman - Medical and Health Encyclopedia (Vol 1-4) - J. G. Fergusan Publishing Co. (1993) Chicago.

7. Brenda Walpale - (vol. 6) Encyciopaedia of Science – MacMillan Publishing Co. (1991), 866 Third Avenue New York.

8. Chressie Wildwood - Creative Aromatherapy - Piatkus Books (1994) 5 Windmill Street, London.

9. Nich. Culpeper - Complete Herbal - Wordsworth Referance (1995) Cumberland House, Crib Street, London.

10. Viktor Blevi and Gretchen Sween - The complete Book of Beauty – Avon Books. (1993) Adiv off- The Hearst Corporation, 1350, Avenue of Americas, New York.

11. Dr. S. K. Jain - Medicinal Plants - National Book Trust, (1994), A-5, Green Park, New Delhi.

12. .Julia Lawless - Home Aromatherapy - Readers Digest, (1993)

13. Maggie Tisserand - Aromabeauty Plan - Vermilion, (1994) Random House, 20 Vauxhall Bridge Road, London.

14. Jill Nice - Herbal Remedies & Home Comforts - Orient Paper Backs (1994), Madarasa Road, Kashmere gate, Delhi-6.

15. Jane Buckle- Clinical Aromatherapy- Churchill Livingstone (2003),

16. David G. Williams- The Chemistry of Essential oils- Micelle Press (1996) 12 Ullswater Crescent, Weymouth, Dorset DT3 5HE.

Dr. RATAN recommends

Eco-Harvested Essential Oils

from

Fm's Aromatherapy

(Aromatantra)

Suppliers of :

- Natural Essential Oils in Retail / Bulk Packing.

- Cold Pressed Base Oils.

- Natural Evening Primrose Oil (10% + GLA)

- Dr. Ratan's Formulations for -

- Skin, Hair & Health Care.

- Range of Wellness Oils

- Chakra Ointments.

- Chakra Crystals / Wands

- Other Healing Crystals / Yantras.

- Dr. Ratan's Books, Cds & DVDs.

For further details & orders contact :

fmsaroma@yahoo.co.uk / aromatantra@yahoo.com

www.fmaromatherapy.com / www.aromatantra.com